ISCHEMIC HEART DISEASE

Edited by **David C. Gaze**

Ischemic Heart Disease
http://dx.doi.org/10.5772/56147
Edited by David C. Gaze

Contributors

Junichi Taki, Magda Youssef, Karina M. Mata, Fabio Carmona, Marcela S. Oliveira, Simone G. Ramos, Anastasia Susie Mihailidou, Rebecca Ritchie, Anthony Ashton, Nadegda Pozdnyakova, Suli Zhang, Jin Wang, Yunhui Du, Jianyu Shang, Li Wang, Jie Wang, Ke Wang, Kehua Bai, Tingting Lv, Xiao Li, Huirong Liu, Guijing Wang, Yigang Wang, Ghulam Naroo, David Gaze

Published by InTech

Janeza Trdine 9, 51000 Rijeka, Croatia

Publishing Process Manager Danijela Duric
Technical Editor InTech DTP team
Cover InTech Design team

Additional hard copies can be obtained from orders@intechopen.com

Ischemic Heart Disease, Edited by David C. Gaze
p. cm.
ISBN 978-953-51-0993-8

For EU product safety concerns:
IN TECH d.o.o., Prolaz Marije Krucifikse Kozulić 3, 51000 Rijeka, Croatia,
info@intechopen.com or visit our website at intechopen.com.

Meet the editor

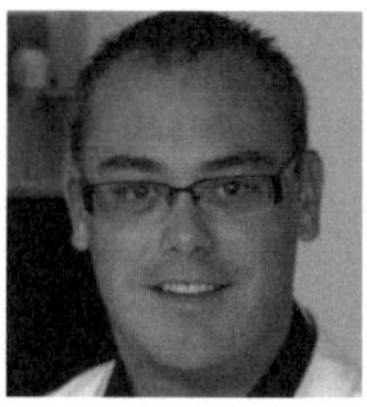

Following undergraduate and postgraduate study in the North of England and London respectively, David Gaze works as a Research Biochemist in the department of Chemical Pathology, Clinical Blood Sciences at St George's Hospital and Medical School, London. His area of research interest is the development and clinical utility of cardiovascular biomarkers for assessment of patients with cardiovascular disease and cardiorenal disease. He has authored and co authored over 130 peer reviewed original papers, editorials and reviews, 150 conference proceedings. In addition, he has authored a number of book chapters, edited works on cardiovascular disease and written a textbook on cardiac troponin. He has delivered national and international presentations on cardiac biomarkers. He received two NACB distinguished abstracts awards (2006/2008) and a diploma for oral presentation from the 17th IFCC–FESCC European Congress of Clinical Chemistry and Laboratory Medicine. He is a member of the American Association of Clinical Biochemistry; Member of the Association for Biochemistry; Associate member of the Royal Institute; Member of the Institute of Biomedical Sciences; Fellow of the Royal Society of Medicine and a member of the Pathological Society of Great Britain.

Contents

Preface

Cardiovascular disease is ranked as the leading cause of death world wide. According to the World Heart Federation, cardiovascular disease is responsible for 17.1 million deaths globally each year. A staggering 82% of these deaths actually occur in the developing world. Such numbers are often difficult to comprehend. The gravity of the situation is enhanced when portrayed as the following: A coronary even occurs every 25 seconds and CHD kills one person every 34 seconds in the United States of America alone. 35 people under the age of 65 die prematurely in the United Kingdom every day due to cardiovascular disease (12,500 deaths per annum). Although the leading killer, the incidence of cardiovascular disease has declined in recent years due to a better understanding of the pathological mechanisms involved and development of targeted therapeutics; along with the implementation of lipid lowering therapy such as statins and new drug regimens including low molecular weight heparin and antiplatelet drugs such as glycoprotein IIb/IIIa receptor inhibitors. Recent advances in acute surgical intervention have also improved mortality, especially with the advent of drug eluting stents and minimally invasive coronary artery bypass grafting, along with improvements in cardioplegia and a systemic hypothermic environment.

The disease burden has a great financial impact on global healthcare systems and major economic consequences for world economies. Cardiovascular disease cost the UK healthcare system £14.4 billion (€16.7 billion; $22.8 billion) in 2006. Hospital care for patients with cardiovascular disease accounts for approximately 70% of the cost with 20% spent on pharmacological agents. The total cost should include non-healthcare costs such as production losses in the workforce and informal care of people with the disease. Production loss is estimated to cost the UK economy £8.2 billion in 2006 (55% due to death and 45% due to illness). Informal care cost the UK economy £8.0 billion in 2006. Overall cardiovascular disease is estimated to cost the UK economy £30.7 billion per annum.

This text firstly introduces the heart and circulation and the development and anatomy of the coronary arteries before introducing the all encompassing umbrella of cardiovascular disease and the Pathobiology of ischemic heart disease (IHD). The epidemiological burden of Ischemic heart disease is described on a global scale; followed by risk factors, diagnostic modalities and treatment regimens for IHD. The next chapter describes the deleterious effects of congenital heart diseases and the role of myocardial ischemia in these conditions, detailing the pathogenesis, diagnosis and treatment options before tacking strategies for prevention. Chapter three demonstrates the gender disparity in sudden cardiac death (SCD). SCD occurs predominantly in women often without previous symptoms or history of CVD. The mechanisms surrounding SCD are detailed followed by identification of those at risk and potential treatment strategies such as implantable cardioverter-defibrillators for high risk subjects. Chapter four reports on the significance of endothelial function and its relationship to silent myocardial ischemia, especially in patients with concomitant diabetes mellitus. Damage to the endothelium is considered to be the initiation of the atherothrombotic episode; be it chemically induced by reduction in nitric oxide, oxidative stress or inflammation or by mechanical sheer stress and hemodynamic disruption. This is followed by the presentation of clinical findings in sixty patients with CHD and type II diabetes Mellitus compared to sixty eight patients with CHD but no evidence of diabetes. Using Holter ECG monitoring, echocardiography, vascular Doppler ultrasound, the vascular responses between those with and those without diabetes were measured. Furthermore, cerebrovascular reactivity testing was also assessed. Patients with CHD and concomitant diabetes demonstrate reduced endothelium-dependent vasodilation compared to those CHD patients without CHD. As mentioned above, the economic cost of CHD is crippling healthcare budgets and contributes to loss of business revenue and national reduction in gross domestic product. Chapter five from experts at the Centers for Disease Control and Prevention, USA surveyed inpatient admissions between 2006-8. Some 41,546 claims were made for a primary diagnosis of acute myocardial infarction (46% ST segment elevation MI; STEMI). The associated costs are highest in males than females and a geographical variation was observed. STEMI costs were higher than non-STEMI costs and costs were highest in those undergoing surgical revascularisation by primary coronary intervention or coronary artery bypass grafting. These data could be used to model more cost-effective AMI intervention programs. The next chapter details the biochemical tests available for the detection and diagnosis of cardiac ischemia. There are a plethora of candidate biomarkers however very few have made the transition to use in the clinical setting. Biomarkers up stream of the cardiac troponins may serve as sensitive tests, but at the cost of specificity thus reducing the overall diagnostic efficiency of the test. Malondialdehyde low-density lipoprotein, Myeloperoxidase, whole blood choline, and free fatty acids are described. The FDA cleared Ischemia Modified Albumin assay is described in detail including its clinical utility not only in acute chest pain but in those patients without acute coronary syndrome. Lastly, with the advent of sensitive cardiac troponin tests, the ischemia vs necrosis debate is challenged once again. Chapter seven discusses the role of uric acid (the end product of purine metabolism) as a risk factor for the development of CVD. Similarly, the role of magnesium and the hypomagnesaemic state and its relationship in the development of clinical disorders such as diabetes, hypertension, atherosclerosis and acute coronary syndrome are discussed in the subsequent chapter. Chapter nine investigates the process of 'self-eating' or autophagy, detailing the intracellular signalling control mechanisms and its role in the maintenance of normal myocardial tissue and its cardioprotective effect during ischemia in the hypoxic myocardium. The understanding of autophagy may lead to possible therapeutic targets for IHD. The penultimate chapter is concerned with progenitor and stem cell engineering as a possible intervention to treat IHD. This is of great interest given recent advances in understanding progenitor cell biology but also poses many considerable challenges in transferring from laboratory based science into a clinical reality. The chapter reviews recent progress in progenitor and stem cell engineering, including cell sources, scaffold free tissue construct, myocardial tissue generation using decellularised native tissue, porous scaffolding and biosynthetic polymers. The final chapter of this text discuses the role of fatty acid imaging, in which fatty acid tracers labelled with the radioisotope of iodine, 123-I is used in single positron emission computer tomography (SPECT) imaging. An overview of myocardial fatty acid metabolism is given, along with description of the iodine-labelled tracers and their myocardial tissue kinetics. This is followed by the clinical utility of the tracer in imaging post acute myocardial infarction, in those with stable chronic coronary artery disease, risk stratification and the assessment of myocardial tissue viability and probably most importantly, prediction of functional recovery. Furthermore, its role in chronic kidney disease is discussed in light of the high prevalence of CHD in this unique population.

David C. Gaze
Dept of Chemical Pathology Clinical Blood Sciences,
St George's Healthcare NHS Trust
London, United Kingdom

Chapter 1

Introduction to Ischemic Heart Disease

David C. Gaze

Additional information is available at the end of the chapter

http://dx.doi.org/10.5772/55248

1. Introduction

"The heart has its reasons which reason knows not." Blaise Pascal (1623-1662)

The heart is the vital organ that tirelessly pumps oxygenated blood from the lungs to the organs and peripheral tissues via the circulatory system. In return, deoxygenated blood is returned via the heart and the pulmonary circulation to the lungs to expel waste carbon dioxide (figure 1). The average human heart beats approximately 72 beats per minute totalling around 2.5 billion beats in a 66-year lifespan. The human heart weighs 250-300g in females and 300-350g in males. The heart is located in the mediastinum of the thorax, anterior to the vertebrae and posterior to the sternum. *Archosaurs* (crocodilians and birds) as well as *Mammalia* species show complete separation of the heart into two pumping units comprised of four distinct chambers. The myogenic musculature of the heart is supplied by the coronary arteries and the entire organ is held within the pericardial sac.

1.1. Development and anatomy of the coronary arteries

As with any organ, the heart requires its own supply of blood for continued functioning. The supply of blood to the myocardium occurs via the coronary artery circuit (figure 2). Their name is derived from the Latin 'Corona', meaning crown as the main vessels encircle the interventricular and atrioventricular grooves.

The arterial tree has two main compartments; firstly, the main arteries (table 1) and ramifications on the surface of the myocardium, known as the extramural coronary system. Secondly, the branches of the surface vessels which penetrate deep into the myocardial tissues are known as the intramural coronary system.

The extramural coronary system is formed from two main arteries. The left coronary artery (LCA) and the right coronary artery (RCA). A third vessel exists in up to 50% of the population and is known as the conus artery. The diameters of the vessels are given in table 1. The intramural coronary system is a complex vascular network containing the main intramural branches which have region specific distribution patterns. The ventricular branches arise at right angles from the subepicardial arteries taking an endocardial route. An important component of the intramural system is the collateral or anastomotic arterial system. These vessels have a characteristic corkscrew appearance. They are present at birth and do not differ in distribution by age or gender. In the normal heart they are 20-350 μm in diameter.

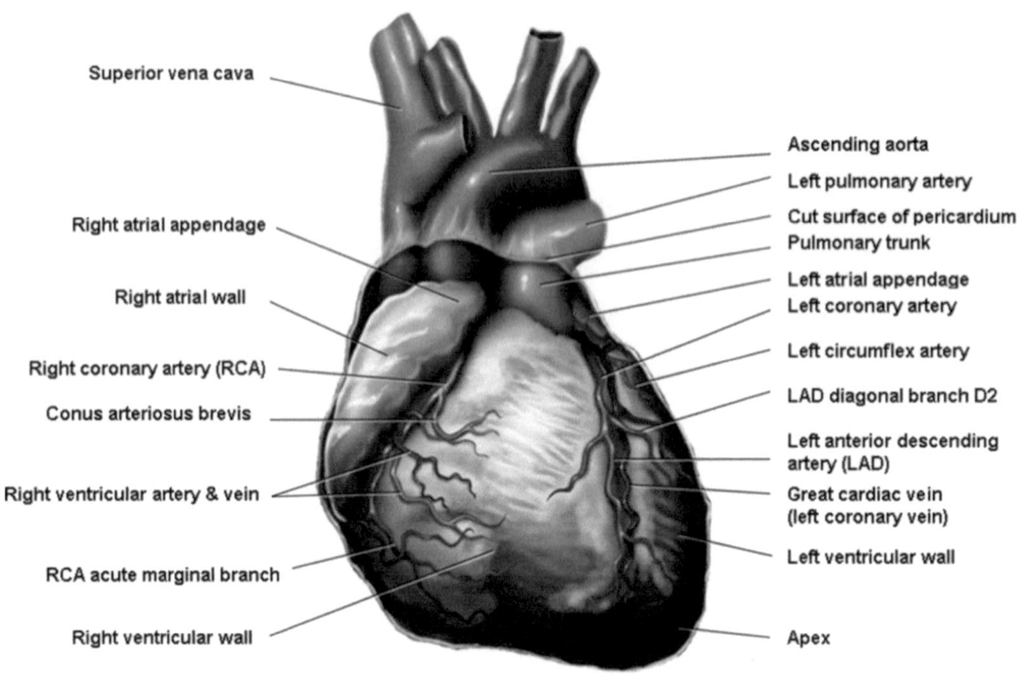

Figure 1. Anterior view of the human heart with blood vessels identified

http://dx.doi.org/10.5772/55248

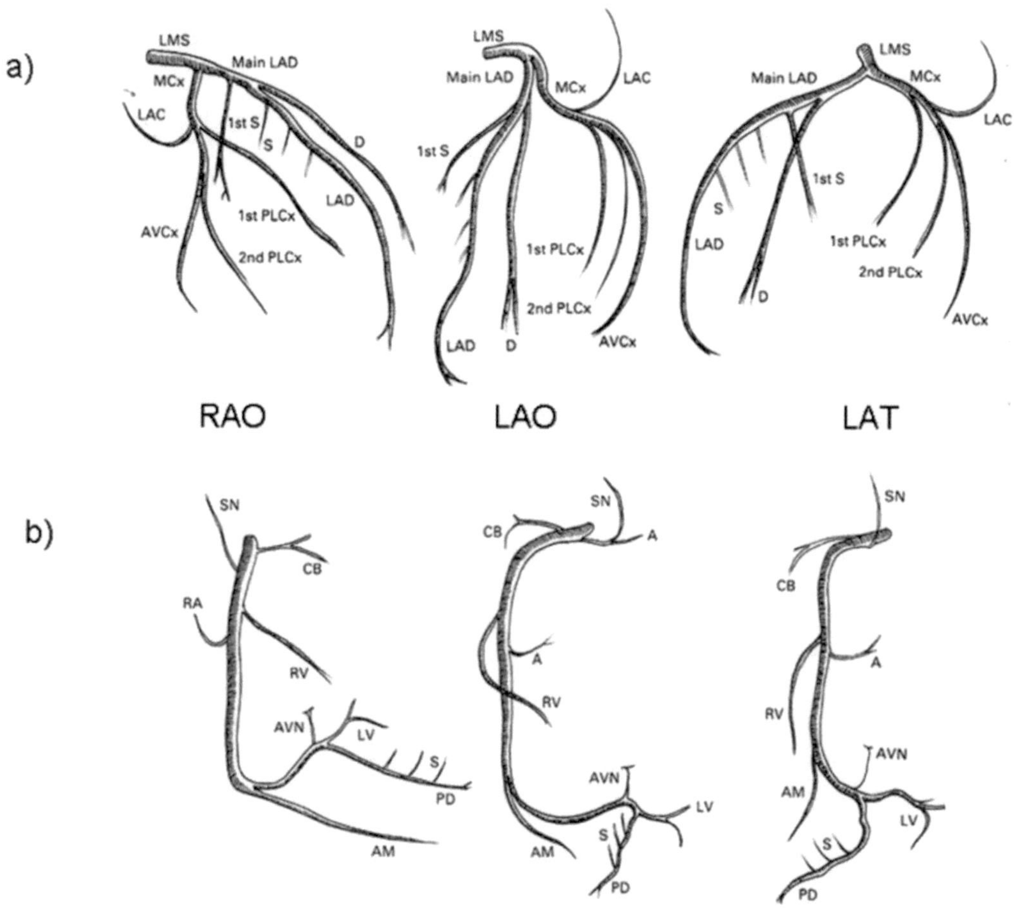

Figure 2. Coronary artery anatomy. a) Left coronary artery and b) Right coronary artery. A, atrial branch; AM, acute marginal artery; AVCx, atrioventricular groove branch of circumflex; AVN, atrioventricular node artery; CB, conus branch; D, diagonal branch of LAD; LAC, left atrial circumflex; LAD, left anterior descending; LAO 30° left anterior oblique projection; LAT, left lateral projection; LMS, left main stem; LV, left ventricular branches; MCx, main circumflex; PD, posterior descending; PLCx, posterior circumflex branch (obtuse marginal); RA, right atrial branch; RAO, 30o right anterior oblique projection; RV, right ventricular branch; S, septal perforating arteries; SN, sinus node artery.

Vessel	Median Diameter (range) in mm
LEFT CORONARY ARTERY (LCA)	4 (2.5-5.5)
Left anterior descending	3.6 (2-5)
DG diagonal	2 (0.5-2.5)
LCX circumflex	3 (1.5-5)
LMG marginal	2.2 (1-3)
RIGHT CORONARY ARTERY (RCA)	3.2 (1.5-5.5)
RMG marginal	1.7 (1-2.5)
PD posterior descending	2.1 (1-3)
THIRD CORONARY ARTERY 'conus artery'	1.1 (0.7-2)
Septal branches anterior from LCX	1 (0.5-2.5)
Septal branches posterior from PD	0.7 (0.3-0.9)
From ascending LAD	0.4 (0.3-0.7)

Table 1. The major coronary arteries.

The primitive embryonic heart is nourished via lacunar or intertrabeclar spaces, forming a net-like structure separating bundles of muscle fibres. Further evolutionary development results in endothelial budding. Originally this was thought to derive from the coronary sinus and aorta, forming superficial veins and arteries which penetrate into the myocardial tissue joining the lacunar spaces. It was then demonstrated in chick-quail chimaeras that the vessels were derived from the proepicardium structure common to the embryo and undergo a transition from epithelial to mesenchymal tissue. Mouse studies refute this, suggesting that the proepicardium gives rise to myocardial stroma and vascular smooth muscle but not coronary artery endothelial cells. Using clonal and histological analysis in the mouse, Red-Horse and colleagues (Red-Horse et al. 2010) demonstrate that coronary arteries are formed by developmental reprogramming of venous cells, arising from angiogenic sprouts of the sinus venosus which returns blood to the embryonic heart. The understanding of angiogenesis in the myocardium may in future lead to more natural methods to stimulate vascular growth and engineering coronary bypass grafts rather than transplanting veins to revascularize damaged myocardium.

2. Cardiovascular disease

A variety of diseases affect the primary functioning of the heart. Cardiovascular disease (CVD) is the collective name for diseases of the heart and blood vessels of the circulatory system. An atlas of types of cardiovascular diseases in the heart and in the circulation are given in table 2.

International efforts have been implemented to classify and code the different types of ischemic heart diseases. A number of notable indexing databases such as the International Classification of Diseases database, Disease Database eMedicine and MeSH databases have produced indexing codes. These are given in table 3.

Cardiovascular Disease	
Diseases of the Heart	**Diseases of the Circulation**
Angina Pectoris	Aortic aneurysm
Stable Angina	
Unstable Angina	Aortitis
Variant (Prinzmetal's) Angina	
	Arteriosclerosis
Arrhythmia	
Heart block (first-degree and second-degree and complete AV block)	Atherosclerosis
Premature atrial complex	
Atrial flutter	Aortic dissection
Paroxysmal supraventricular tachycardia	
Wolff-Parkinson-White syndrome	Hypertension
Premature ventricular complex	Essential (primary) hypertension
Ventricular tachycardia	Secondary hypertension
Ventricaular fibrillation	Malignant hypertension
Long QT syndrome	
	Stroke (Cerebrovascular accident)
Cardiomyopathy	
Dilated Cardiomyopathy	Transient ischemic attack
Hypertropic Cardiomyopathy	
Restrictive Cardiomyopathy	Arterial disease
	Arterial embolus
Congestive heart failure	Acute arterial occlusion
	Raynaud's phenomenon
Congenital heart disease	Arteriovenous fistula
Atrial septal defect	Vasculitis
Ventricular septal defect	Thoracic outlet syndrome
Patent ductus arteriosus	

Cardiovascular Disease	
Diseases of the Heart	**Diseases of the Circulation**
Pulmonary stenosis	Venous disease
Congential aortic stenosis	Venous thrombosis
Teratology of Fallot	Deep vein thrombosis
Tricuspid atresia	Varicose veins
Truncus arteriosus	Spider veins
Ebstein's abnormality of the tricuspid valve	
Great vessel transposition	Lymphedema
Coronary artery disease	
Ischemic heart disease	
Acute myocardial infarction	
Cor pulmonale	
Heart valve disease	
Mitral stenosis	
Mitral valve regurgitation	
Mitral valve prolapse	
Aortic stenosis	
Aortic regurgitation	
Tricuspid stenosis	
Tricuspid regurgitation	
Myocarditis	
Rheumatic disease	
Pericarditis	
Sudden cardiac death	
Syncope	
Cardiac tumours	
Myxoma	

Table 2. Atlas of cardiovascular diseases of the heart and circulatory system.

http://dx.doi.org/10.5772/55248

Classification system	Code	
International Classification of Diseases (ICD-9) World Health Organisation, Geneva, Switzerland	410	Acute Myocardial infarction (AMI)
	411	Other acute and subsequent forms of Ischemic Heart Disease
	412	Old Myocardial Infarction
	413	Angina Pectoris
	414	Other forms of chronic ischemic heart disease
International Classification of Diseases (ICD-10) World Health Organisation, Geneva, Switzerland	120	Angina Pectoris
	121	Acute Myocardial Infarction (AMI)
	122	Subsequent Myocardial Infarction
	123	Certain current complications following AMI
	124	Other acute ischemic heart diseases
	125	Chronic ischemic heart disease
Diseases Database (DiseaseDB) Medical Object Oriented Software Enterprises Ltd London UK	8695 - Ischemic or Ischaemic Heart disease, Myocardial Ischaemia, Steoncardia, Angina Pectoris, Coronary Artery Arteriosclerosis, IHD	
eMedicine (WebMD) New York, USA	Med/1568 – Angina Pectoris	
Medical Subject headings (MeSH) Unites States National Library of Medicine Bethesda, Maryland, USA	D017202 – Myocardial Ischemia	

Table 3. Classification codes of Ischemic Heart Disease

3. Pathobiology of ischemic heart disease

Hypoxia refers to the physiological or pathological state in which oxygen supply is reduced despite adequate perfusion of the tissue. Anoxia is the absence of oxygen from the tissue, despite being adequately perfused. These are clearly distinguishable from ischemia where oxygen supply is restricted as a direct result of suboptimal tissue perfusion. Ischemic tissue also accumulates toxic metabolites due to the inadequate removal through the capillary and venous blood systems.

The atherosclerotic process responsible for restriction of blood flow in the coronary arteries is a multifactorial process and is initiated by damage to the endothelium. Cholesterol rich low density lipoprotein (LDL) particles enter the intimal layer via the LDL receptor protein (Brown and Goldstein 1979), a mosaic cell surface protein that recognizes apolipoprotein B100 embedded in the LDL particle. It also recognizes apolipoprotein E found in chylomicrons and very low density lipoprotein remnants, or intermediate density lipoprotein. Macrophage cells accumulate oxidized lipid independently of the LDL receptor by endocytosis. This results in formation of juvenile raised fatty streaks within the endothelium. The macrophage release their lipid content and cytokines into the intima. Cytokines stimulate intimal thickening by smooth muscle cell proliferation, which then secrete collagen, causing fibrosis (figure 3). The lesion appears raised and yellow.

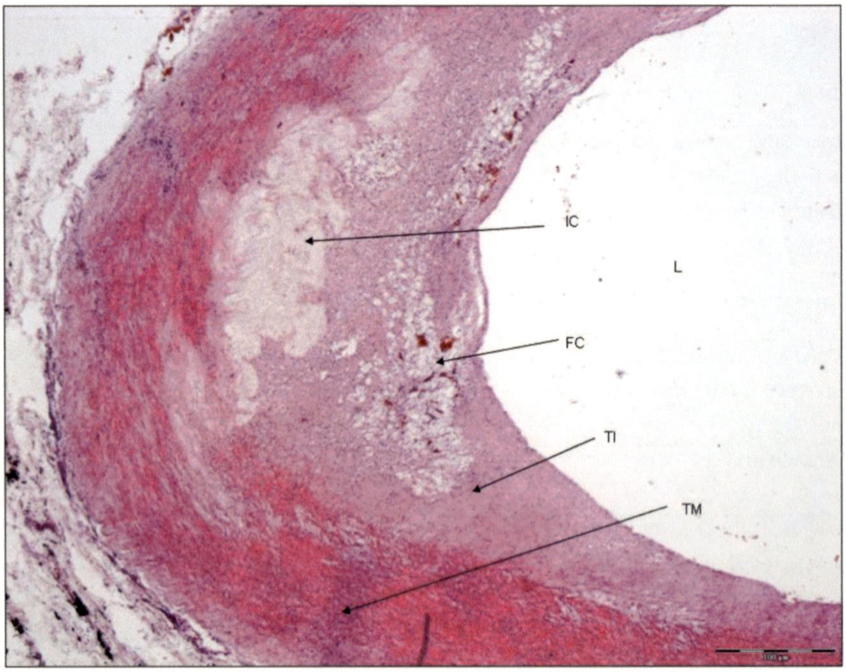

Figure 3. Medium powered H&E histological micrograph of an intimal lesion (x200). FC, foam cell infiltrate; IC, intimal calcification; L, lumen; TI, tunica intima; TM, tunica media.

As the lesion develops, the medial layer of the vessel wall atrophies and the elastic lamina becomes disrupted. Collagen forms a fibrous cap over the lesion that appears hard and white (known as a fibrolipid plaque). The plaque contains macrophage laden with lipid (foam cells) as well as extracellular or 'free' lipid within the lesion. The endothelium is now in a fragile state. Ulceration of the cap occurs at weak points such as the shoulder region, near the endothelial lining. Rupture to the cap can cause turbulent blood flow in the lumen. The exposed lipid core causes aggregation of platelets and development of a thrombosis. This lesion grows due to further platelet aggregation and is responsible for narrowing of the lumen of the artery resulting in localized ischemia. Distal embolization of a piece of such thrombus may travel downstream and can completely occlude smaller arteries.

The symptomatic part of the continuum is known as the acute coronary syndrome (ACS) which is due to the rupture/erosion of the plaque. This produces, depending on the plaque size, vascular anatomy and presence of collateral vessels, a mismatch between the supply and demand for oxygen. A net reduction in supply compared to the demand results in ischemia. Tissue hypoxia proceeds resulting in inadequate blood/oxygen perfusion. If blood flow is not re-established, cardiac cell necrosis will occur. Post AMI survival results in remodelling processes in the myocardium and the development of cardiac failure.

http://dx.doi.org/10.5772/55248

4. Epidemiology of ischemic heart disease

According to the World Health Organisation, chronic diseases of which heart disease is the single largest contributing category; are responsible for 63% of all global deaths (United Nations High-Level Meeting on Noncommunicable Disease Prevention and Control 2012). Non communicable diseases kill 9 million people under the age of 60 every year which has a profound socio-economic impact.

The incidence of Ischemic heart disease (IHD) is higher than for any cancer or other non-CVD condition. Cardiovascular diseases (CVD) are the leading cause of death in the Western World and are dramatically increasing within developing countries. The Age-standardized estimate of mortality by cardiovascular diseases and diabetes per 100,000 people is given in figure 4. 17.1 million people die as a direct result of CVD per year and 82% of these deaths occur in the developing word

It is predicted that by 2030 23 million people will die from a CVD. Data from the USA suggests that CVD was responsible for 34% of deaths in 2006 and over 151,000 Americans who died were <65 years old. The incidence of CVD is declining in the Western World even though rates of lifestyle associated risk factors such as obesity, smoking and type II diabetes mellitus are increasing. The decline is in part due to advances in therapeutic and invasive intervention. In creating better outcomes for those with acute cardiac conditions, patients develop heart failure which requires longer term treatment and monitoring and may in fact be a greater health burden than the acute events themselves.

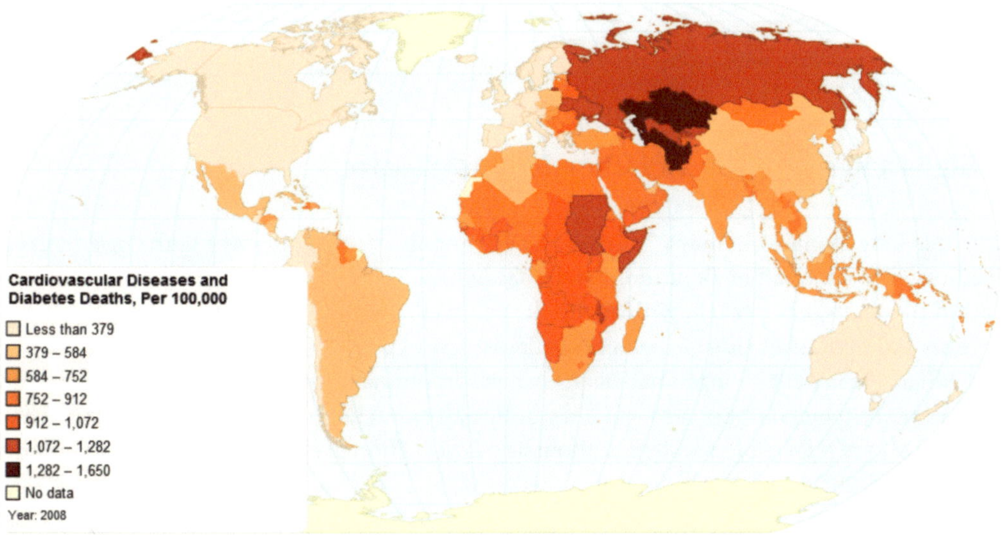

Figure 4. Age-standardized estimate of mortality by cardiovascular diseases and diabetes per 100,000 people. Source: Global Health Observatory Data Repository, World Health Organisation.

5. Risk factors

There is no single causative risk factor for the development of IHD. A number of genetic and environmental risk factors have been established as causative in the development of the atherosclerotic lesion. Smoking and obesity cause 36% and 20% of IHD respectively. A large European meta-analysis of 197,473 participants reported an small association between job stress and the development of coronary artery disease (Kivimaki et al. 2012). There has been extensive research linking a sedentary lifestyle and a lack of exercise with a risk of IHD. The major risk factors for the development of IHD are given in table 4.

Constant risk factors	**Modifiable risk factors**
Age	Hypercholesterolaemia/dyslipidaemia
Gender	Hypertension
Family history of IHD	Obesity (particularly central abdominal obesity)
Personal history of early IHD	Tobacco and passive tobacco Smoking
Diabetes Mellitus type I	Excessive alcohol consumption
Elevated homocysteine	Diabetes Mellitus type II
Elevated haemostatic factors	Sedentary lifestyle
Baldness & hair greying	Low antioxidant levels
Earlobe crease (Frank's sign)	Infection
	Air pollution (CO, NO_2, SO_2)
	Combined oral contraceptive pill

Table 4. Risk factors for the development of Ischaemic Heart Disease.

6. Signs and symptoms of ischemic heart disease

Ischemia may manifest in many forms. Most commonly, patients present with chest pain on exertion, in cold weather or in emotional situations. This discomfort is known as angina pectoris. Patients may present with acute chest pain at rest which typically radiates down the left arm and up the left side of the neck. Patients may experience nausea, vomiting, sweating and enhanced anxiety. Symptomatically, women present with less 'textbook' symptoms and often describe their condition as weakness, indigestion and fatigue (Kosuge et al. 2006). Up to 60% of AMI are referred to as silent without any observation of chest pain or other symptoms (Valensi et al. 2011).

Angina is diagnosed by evidence of deviation of the ST segment on the electrocardiogram, reduced uptake of thallium-201 during myocardial perfusion imaging or regional or global impairment of ventricular function. In patients with stable angina often have chest pain on exertion. Patients benefit from cardiac stress testing, echocardiography. If indicated patients should receive coronary angiography to locate anatomically any stenosis with a view to revascularisation by stenting during percutaneous coronary intervention or coronary artery bypass grafting (CABG) surgery.

7. Diagnosis of ischemic heart disease

In the primary care setting, patients may be suspected of having ischemic heart disease based on risk factor assessment and blood chemistry tests such as lipid profiling, inflammatory markers and homocysteine concentration.

Primarily the diagnosis of IHD occurs in the acute setting when patients present with symptomatic chest pain. Patients often present with a myriad of symptoms which confuse the clinical picture. Patients should receive immediate electrocardiography and pharmacological or surgical intervention in those who demonstrate ST-segment elevation in the context of ST-segment myocardial infarction (STEMI). In suspected non-ST segment elevation myocardial infarction (NSTEMI) patients should undergo serial venepuncture for cardiac biomarkers, namely the cardiac troponins which are indicative of myocyte necrosis. Patients may undergo stress testing, whereby the stress response is induced by exercise or pharmacological agents allowing comparison of the coronary circulation at rest and under stress. Patients are monitored continuously whilst exercising on a treadmill, on a ergometer bicycle or following injection of agents such as adenosine, the adenosine A2A receptor Regadenoson or the beta-agonist dobutamine. The agent of choice is dependent on drug interactions with medication or concomitant disease states.

Cardiac ultrasound or echocardiography by two-dimensional, three-dimensional or Doppler ultrasound create images of the myocardium at work. Transthoracic echocardiogram (TTE) is the commonest form and the ultrasound transducer probe is placed non-invasively on the thorax. Transoesophageal echogram (TOE) is an alternative method where the transducer tip is passed into the oesophagus, allowing imaging directly behind the heart.

8. Treatment of ischemic heart disease

Stable IHD patients can be adequately treated in the primary care setting with emphasis on both lifestyle and risk factor modifications to reduce the risk of a future adverse cardiac event. Modification of lifestyle risk factors such as smoking cessation and weight loss control have a direct impact on risk reduction. Further intervention such as treating hypertension, glycaemic control in diabetics and therapeutic intervention in hyperlipidaemia result in risk reduction. Furthermore, elective revascularisation of occluded coronary arteries may confer a reduction in mortality risk compared to conservative therapy. A meta-analysis of 13,121 patients in whom 6476 were randomised to revascularisation compared to medical treatment in the remainder demonstrated that bypass grafting and Percutaneous coronary intervention are superior to medical therapy alone with respect to 1-10 year mortality (Jeremias et al. 2009).

Patients with symptomatic chest pain suggestive of an AMI and ST segment elevation should receive immediate revascularisation. Fibrinolytic therapy should be administered within 30 minutes and door-to-balloon PCI should occur in no more than 90 minutes from the onset of pain. For non ST segment elevation AMI patients, treatment with aspirin, glycoprotein IIb/IIIa inhibitor such as clopidogrel, low molecular weight heparin, glyceryl trinitrate and opioid therapy for persistent pain.

9. Conclusion

Ischemic heart disease is the major contributing cause of death in the Western World and the incidence is increasing in developing countries. Successful advances in surgical and therapeutic intervention are able to salvage myocardial tissue and increase prognosis if administered in the early phase following injury.

Author details

David C. Gaze

Department of Chemical Pathology Clinical Blood Sciences, St. George's Healthcare NHS Trust, London, UK

References

[1] Brown, M. S, & Goldstein, J. L. (1979). Receptor-mediated endocytosis: insights from the lipoprotein receptor system. *Proc.Natl.Acad.Sci.U.S.A* , 76, 3330-3337.

[2] Jeremias, A, Kaul, S, Rosengart, T. K, Gruberg, L, & Brown, D. L. (2009). The impact of revascularization on mortality in patients with nonacute coronary artery disease. *Am.J.Med.* , 122, 152-161.

[3] Kivimaki, M, Nyberg, S. T, Batty, G. D, Fransson, E. I, Heikkila, K, Alfredsson, L, Bjorner, J. B, Borritz, M, Burr, H, Casini, A, Clays, E, De Bacquer, D, Dragano, N, Ferrie, J. E, Geuskens, G. A, Goldberg, M, Hamer, M, Hooftman, W. E, Houtman, I. L, Joensuu, M, Jokela, M, Kittel, F, Knutsson, A, Koskenvuo, M, Koskinen, A, Kouvonen, A, Kumari, M, Madsen, I. E, Marmot, M. G, Nielsen, M. L, Nordin, M, Oksanen, T, Pentti, J, Rugulies, R, Salo, P, Siegrist, J, Singh-manoux, A, Suominen, S. B, Vaananen, A, Vahtera, J, Virtanen, M, Westerholm, P. J, Westerlund, H, Zins, M, Steptoe, A,

& Theorell, T. (2012). Job strain as a risk factor for coronary heart disease: a collaborative meta-analysis of individual participant data. *Lancet* , 380, 1491-1497.

[4] Kosuge, M, Kimura, K, Ishikawa, T, Ebina, T, Hibi, K, Tsukahara, K, Kanna, M, Iwahashi, N, Okuda, J, Nozawa, N, Ozaki, H, Yano, H, Nakati, T, Kusama, I, & Umemura, S. (2006). Differences between men and women in terms of clinical features of ST-segment elevation acute myocardial infarction. *Circ.J.* , 70, 222-226.

[5] Red-horse, K, Ueno, H, Weissman, I. L, & Krasnow, M. A. (2010). Coronary arteries form by developmental reprogramming of venous cells. *Nature* , 464, 549-553.

[6] United Nations High-Level Meeting on Noncommunicable Disease Prevention and Control. (2012).

[7] Valensi, P, Lorgis, L, & Cottin, Y. (2011). Prevalence, incidence, predictive factors and prognosis of silent myocardial infarction: a review of the literature. *Arch.Cardiovasc.Dis.* , 104, 178-188.

Chapter 2

Myocardial Ischemia in Congenital Heart Disease: A Review

Fabio Carmona, Karina M. Mata,
Marcela S. Oliveira and Simone G. Ramos

Additional information is available at the end of the chapter

http://dx.doi.org/10.5772/53420

1. Introduction

1.1. Concepts

Patients with congenital heart disease (CxHD) are surviving into adulthood, as well as living longer and growing older [1], due the major achievements in their diagnosis, medical management, surgical repair, and postoperative treatment in the last three to four decades. An increasing numbers of patients with CxHD are encountered in our everyday practice. It is therefore timely and appropriate to start addressing the somewhat-neglected issue of myocardial ischemia in this patient population [2].

CxHD is, by definition, cardiovascular disease present at birth. It refers to anatomic defects and gross cardiac abnormalities due to an embryologic malformation in the structural development of the heart and major blood vessels, which is actually of functional significance [3]. Most CxHD occur due to gross structural developmental cardiovascular anomalies such as septal defects, stenosis or atresia of valves, hypoplasia or absence of one ventricle, or abnormal connections between great vessels and the heart. A few children are also born with arrhythmias (mainly conduction defects), and hypertrophic or dilated cardiomyopathy, although these are usually present later in childhood or adulthood. CxHD are the most common of all congenital malformations, with a reported incidence of 6 to 8 cases per 1,000 live births, and in an even higher percentage of foetuses [4]. In some studies this incidence reaches 12 to 14 per 1,000 live births [5].

There is a great number of recognized heart defects occurring alone and in combination, ranging in severity from hemodynamically insignificant to extremely complex and life threatening conditions (Table 1). Although there may be genetic or environmental situations that can affect the development of heart defects, in the majority of cases the cause is considered multifactorial, with no specific identifiable trigger. Only approximately 15% of cases of CxHD can be traced to a known cause [6]. Some types of CxHD can be related to chromosome or gene defects, environmental factors or a multifactorial aetiology [7]. Only 2% of all cases of CxHD can be attributed to known environmental factors. Risk factors, such as maternal insulin-dependent diabetes mellitus and phenylketonuria, are well known as two of the leading causes of CxHD. Other reported risk factors include maternal obesity, alcohol use in pregnancy, rubella infection, febrile illness, use of drugs such as thalidomide and retinoic acid, and exposure to organic solvents and lithium [8].

• Patent ductus arteriosus	• Interrupted aortic arch
• Atrial septal defect	• Hypoplastic left heart syndrome
• Ventricular septal defect	• d-Transposition of the great arteries
• Atrioventricular septal defect	• l-Transposition of the great arteries (also known as congenitally-corrected transposition of the great arteries)
• Aortopulmonary window	• Truncus arteriosus communis
• Tetralogy of Fallot	• Double outlet right or left ventricle
• Pulmonary atresia or stenosis	• Ebstein's disease
• Aortic atresia or stenosis	• Anomalies of the coronary arteries
• Mitral atresia or stenosis	• Vascular rings and pulmonary sling
• Tricuspid atresia or stenosis	• Total or partial anomalous pulmonary venous connection
• Left ventricular outflow obstruction	
• Coarctation of the aorta	

Table 1. Most common types of congenital heart defects.

Mortality occurs mainly in patients with severe forms of CxHD requiring prompt surgical intervention [9]. Interestingly, the relative contribution of the causes of death in patients with CxHD has changed over time. The CxHD causes 3% of all infant deaths and 46% of death from congenital malformations, despite advances in detection and treatment. Arrhythmia followed by congestive heart failure had been considered the main contributing cause of death. However, the mortality figures collected over the past decade showed an increase in myocardial infarction as the cause of death [10]. Until the twentieth century, the majority of newborns with CxHD died because treatment was not available. With the advances made in the field of foetal and paediatric cardiology, survival and quality of life have improved, especially in the past 10–20 years [11].

1.2. Myocardial ischemia

The advances in paediatric cardiac surgery were accompanied by refinements in extracorporeal perfusion technology that have led to significant improvements in the surgical results during the past decades. Nevertheless, perioperative myocardial damage still remains the most common cause of morbidity and death after a technically successful surgical correction.

Despite the importance of this issue, there are a few publications about this. Studies show that the younger the age of patients, the more vulnerable are their myocardium to injury caused by ischemia during definitive repair of congenital heart disease. Therefore, perioperative care for paediatric patients with congenital heart disease needs to take into consideration the dependence of the myocardial damage on age and ischemic time [12]. Others researches have shown that myocardial cell injury in infants submitted to open-heart surgery can be directly associated with varying combinations of gross, microscopic, and histochemical myocardial necrosis in up to 90% of patients who do not survive the perioperative period. The observed alterations within the myocardium can potentially be attributed to the heart defect itself, preoperative hemodynamic instability and its treatment, surgical techniques, cardiopulmonary bypass, myocardial protection strategies, and postoperative medical care.

Furthermore, patients with CxHD are at increased risk of developing myocardial ischemia or premature coronary artery disease (CAD) as the result of: (a) congenital coronary artery abnormalities (e.g., anomalous origin and course of coronary arteries, myocardial bridging, coronary artery fistulas); (b) previous surgery (e.g., arterial switch operation for d-transposition of the great arteries (d-TGA) and surgical coarctation repair); and (c) myocardial ischemia not related directly to coronary artery anomalies but presenting after the atrial switch procedure for TGA (Mustard, Senning) and also in patients with congenitally corrected transposition of the great arteries (ccTGA).

Clinical suspicion is a difficult task, especially in neonates and young infants, in whom the clinical manifestations can be unspecific and transient. In older children and adolescents, chest pain can be present, although myocardial ischemia is rarely the underlying cause [13].

The diagnostic and treatment of paediatric CxHD has undergone remarkable progress over the last 60 years [14]. Moreover, in the past 10 years, significant advancements have been made in foetal echocardiography; in postnatal echocardiography and angiography, leading to greater accuracy in defining the cardiac defect; in interventional catheterization as a palliative or curative measure; and in surgical techniques, which have led to an estimated million adults living today with complex CxHD that required surgery in the neonatal period [15].

In the long term, as a consequence of successful cardiac surgeries in the past decades, there is an increasing number of patients with CxHD reaching adulthood and becoming old. These survivors with complex heart defects are now developing problems associated with aging. The association of CxHD, heart surgeries, and chronic coronary artery disease is not well studied yet [16]. It is possible that these patients are at an increased risk of myocardial ischemia, but epidemiological studies are needed to answer to this question.

Therefore, perioperative myocardial injury is a major determinant of cardiac dysfunction after operations for CxHD. It is very important detect and evaluate the degree of myocardial injury as soon as possible after the operative procedure. Thus in an attempt to clarify possible mechanisms involved in the development of ischemic heart disease in children with CxHD, this study aims to describe the pathological alterations observed in different types of CxHD in the heart of infants submitted to surgical correction of cardiac malformations, and to discuss potential strategies to prevent them.

2. Pathogenesis

In normal conditions, an uninterrupted flow of large quantities of oxygenated blood to the myocardium is critical to its normal function [17]. During the systole, this flow can be abolished or even reversed towards the epicardial vessels. The blood must flow from low to high intra-myocardial pressure, in order to meet the metabolic demands of each layer. Such flow must be regulated in such way that areas of high demand can immediately increase their blood supply.

The myocardium extracts about 60 to 75% of oxygen from the blood that passes through it. Because of this high level of extraction, coronary sinus blood has low oxygen tension, generally around 25–35 mm Hg. This low level of oxygen tension requires that any increase in oxygen demand be met by an increase in blood flow rather than an increase in extraction [17].

There are two main mechanisms by which myocardial ischemia can occur: (a) a reduction in myocardial supply of oxygen, and (b) an increase in myocardial oxygen demand [18]. The first situation can occur as a result of reduced coronary blood flow or reduced oxygen content despite normal coronary flow. A reduced coronary blood flow can result from congenital malformations of the coronary arteries, acquired coronary diseases, and also postoperative states, especially after surgical reimplantation of the coronary arteries. Examples of reduced oxygen content in coronary blood include cyanotic heart diseases, severe anaemia, and hemoglobinopathies. The second mechanism can occur in the presence of hypertrophic cardiomyopathy or vigorous exercises. The main diagnoses related to myocardial ischemia are summarized in Table 2.

A number of conditions can lead to myocardial ischemia, including prenatal and birth conditions, the anatomic defect, pre- and postoperative care, surgical technique, and myocardial protection during CPB. These conditions will be discussed in detail below.

2.1. Prenatal and birth conditions

Foetal hearts show a remarkable ability to develop under hypoxic conditions. The metabolic flexibility of foetal hearts allows sustained development under low oxygen conditions. In fact, hypoxia is critical for proper myocardial formation [19]. However, although "normal" hypoxia (lower oxygen tension in the foetus as compared with the adult) is essential in heart formation, further abnormal hypoxia in utero adversely affects cardiogenesis. Prenatal hypoxia alters myocardial structure and causes a decline in cardiac performance. Not only are the effects of hypoxia apparent during the perinatal period, but prolonged hypoxia in utero also causes foetal programming of abnormality in the heart's development. The altered expression patterns of cardioprotective genes likely predispose the developing heart to increased vulnerability to ischemia and reperfusion injury later in life [19].

In addition, myocardial dysfunction is a frequent sequel of perinatal asphyxia, resulting from hypoxic-ischemic damage to the myocardium. It can lead to decreased perfusion, tachycardia, hypotension, and need for inotropic support [20,21]. As a consequence, hemodynamic

Diagnosis related to the coronary arteries
• Anomalous coronary arteries
• Left main coronary artery from the pulmonary artery • Left main coronary from the right coronary cusp • Right coronary artery from the left coronary cusp
• Coronary artery fistula • Coronary artery spasm • Thromboembolic or embolic coronary artery disease • Kawasaki disease • Coronary artery dissection • Ostial coronary artery disease status post surgical reimplantation
• d-Transposition of the great arteries (d-TGA) arterial switch • Aortic root replacement • Ross procedure
• Intramyocardial bridging
Diagnosis related to the myocardium (supply/demand mismatch)
• Hypertrophic cardiomyopathy • Severe aortic stenosis • Dilated cardiomyopathy • Tachycardia in the face of limited coronary blood flow
Others
• Severe hypoxia or cyanosis

Table 2. Diagnosis related to myocardial ischemia.

impairment can develop and the myocardium may suffer additional ischemic insults. Infections, need for cardiopulmonary resuscitation, mechanical ventilation, preterm birth, among other factors may also contribute to myocardial damage during this period.

2.2. The anatomic defect

Many CxHD are associated with anomalies such that the child is prone to myocardial ischemia even after uncomplicated delivery and good hemodynamic conditions. They involve congenital anomalies of the coronary arteries and hypertrophic cardiomyopathy. Other diseases can present early in life with congestive heart failure, circulatory shock, or severe hypoxemia. All these factors can compromise coronary circulation and lead to myocardial ischemia.

2.2.1. Congenital anomalies of the coronary arteries

The entire blood flow to the myocardium comes from two main coronary arteries that arise from the right and left aortic sinuses of Valsalva. In 69% of the population, the right coronary artery is dominant [18]. Although there are normal variations for the coronary anatomy, a comprehensive discussion of this topic is beyond the scope of this chapter, which will focus only on the clinically significant anomalies.

The most common anomaly, accounting for about one third of all major coronary arterial anomalies, is origin of the left circumflex coronary artery from the right main coronary artery. However, this anomaly is rarely of clinical significance. Less common, the origin of the left coronary artery from the right sinus of Valsalva, is of greater significance, and was associated with sudden death in children during or just after vigorous exercise when the vessel passes between the two great arteries [18].

A single coronary artery may be observed in 5–20% of major coronary anomalies. About 40% of these anomalies are associated with other cardiac malformations, including d-TGA, tetralogy of Fallot, ccTGA, double-inlet left ventricle, double-outlet right ventricle, truncus arteriosus, coronary-cameral fistulas, and bicuspid aortic valve [18]. Only a small number of premature deaths have been reported with this anomaly.

When the coronary arteries (either right or left) have their origins in inappropriate sinus, the mechanism of ischemia and death involves an increase in myocardial oxygen demand during exercise that, in turn, causes increases in systolic blood pressure and aortic root distension. If part of the anomalous artery runs within or adjacent to the aortic wall, it may be stretched, compressed, or both, leading to insufficient coronary blood flow.

Other rare coronary anomalies include coronary atresia, stenosis or atresia of a coronary ostium, all coronary arteries from pulmonary artery, left anterior descending coronary artery from pulmonary artery, left circumflex coronary artery from the pulmonary artery or branches, right coronary artery from pulmonary artery, myocardial bridges, etc.

2.2.2. Anomalous origin of left coronary artery from the pulmonary artery (ALCAPA)

In this anomaly the left coronary artery arises from the pulmonary artery. Therefore, after birth, the left ventricle is perfused with desaturated blood in a regimen of low pressures. The left ventricle becomes then hypoxic, and collaterals start to develop. The left ventricle vessels then dilate to reduce their resistance and increase flow, but this is often not enough to prevent ischemia with compromise of the left ventricular function. This leads to congestive heart failure that can be worsened by mitral regurgitation. With time, the collaterals between right and left coronary artery enlarge until the collateral flow tends to reverse in the left coronary and ultimately into the pulmonary artery. The left-to-right shunt is usually not significant [18,22].

This anomaly is usually isolated but can be associated with patent ductus arteriosus, ventricular septal defect, tetralogy of Fallot, or coarctation of the aorta [18].

2.2.3. Tetralogy of fallot

In this disease, a hypertrophied right ventricle is always present, with a high oxygen demand to overcome the outflow tract obstruction and provide pulmonary blood flow. In face of severe cyanosis, hemodynamic impairment, the oxygen supply may not balance the high requirements of the right ventricle, leading to myocardial ischemia.

2.2.4. Pulmonary atresia with intact ventricular septum

In this disease, the absence of anterograde blood flow across the pulmonary valve associated with the absence of a ventricular septal defect precludes the development of the right ventricle, which becomes hypoplastic. A network of vascular channels, called sinusoids, then develops, communicating the right ventricular cavity with one or both of the coronary arteries.

With systemic or supra-systemic systolic pressure within the right ventricular cavity, blood flow in these fistulous connections may compete with the normal coronary blood flow originating in the ascending aorta. Sometimes, these competing blood coronary streams may cause tortuosity, severe intimal proliferation with obstruction, such that portions of the myocardium may be dependent on the right ventricle-originated coronary flow (so-called right ventricle-dependent coronary circulation) [23]. This portion of the myocardium would then be perfused with unsaturated blood. If these sinusoids are not diagnosed properly, a pulmonary valvotomy can be catastrophic, since the sudden fall in right ventricle pressure will reflect in a dramatic fall in coronary pressure, leading to acute myocardial ischemia and, potentially, death.

2.2.5. Other heart defects

Children with a large patent ductus arteriosus with left-to-right shunt, those with severe aortic regurgitation, and those with hypoplastic left heart syndrome, among others, are at great risk for myocardial ischemia, especially in the presence of severe hypoxemia or hypotension. A large patent ductus arteriosus with significant left-to-right shunt can decrease the diastolic pressure in the aorta, significantly diminishing coronary blood flow. A severe aortic regurgitation can lead the same deleterious consequences in diastolic pressure. In patients with hypoplastic left heart syndrome, the ascending aorta receives a retrograde poorly oxygenated blood flow originated from a patent ductus arteriosus. Therefore, these patients are particularly sensitive to hypotension, severe hypoxemia, imbalances between pulmonary and systemic blood flows, and a claudicating ductus arteriosus.

In patients with ccTGA, the right ventricle supports the systemic circulation and can become dilated and hypertrophied with time. Once ventricular dilation and hypertrophy settle in, the blood supply through a normal right coronary artery can become insufficient to meet the increased metabolic demands of the systemic right ventricle [24,25], leading to further ventricular dysfunction. The latter may also have a deleterious effect on left ventricular perfusion, ultimately leading to left ventricular dysfunction [24]. Hypertrophy can also develop in many other situations, especially aortic stenosis and chronic systemic hypertension.

2.3. Preoperative care and drugs

Preoperative care is of special interest in neonates and young infants because usually the CxHD manifests as a critical illness. The neonatal myocardium is less compliant than that of the older child, is less tolerant to increases in afterload, and is less responsive to increases in preload. In the other hand, despite being more labile, this age group is more resilient to metabolic or ischemic injuries, which can play a relative protective role [17]. After birth, neonates with CxHD can deteriorate their hemodynamic status requiring prompt interventions. The higher metabolic rate and oxygen consumption of the neonate account for the rapid appearance of hypoxemia in this age group. In addition, undiagnosed infants and older children may present in shock, congestive heart failure, severe hypoxemia, severe arrhythmia with hemodynamic impairment, or a combination of them, also requiring immediate intensive care. This highly specialized care requires careful evaluation of the structure and function of the heart, the transitional neonatal circulation, and the secondary effects of the defect on other organ systems. All efforts need to be put on making a definitive, precise diagnosis, so appropriate therapeutic measures can be started [17].The treatment of the newborn or infant with severe hemodynamic compromise often involves the use of catecholamines that, despite improving myocardial contractility, can further increase the myocardial metabolic rate and oxygen consumption. Therefore, the attending clinician shall be aware that these drugs need to be used only at the minimum effective dose to obtain the desired effect. Alternatively, when the renal function is preserved, milrinone and levosimendan are very good options, since they can increase myocardial contractility without increasing metabolic rate and oxygen consumption.

Special attention shall be put also on coronary blood flow. Careful monitoring with continuous electrocardiography, as well as serially measuring CK-MB and cardiac troponins, is mandatory for the child with severe hemodynamic impairment, and prompt interventions need to be done quickly in face of a suspected or confirmed coronary insufficiency.

In older patients, the CxHD usually present as congestive heart failure or arrhythmias, not requiring critical care before surgery. There are, obviously, exceptions that shall be properly managed.

2.4. Surgical technique

2.4.1. d-Transposition of the great arteries

In this malformation, a number of different patterns of coronary anatomy have been described. Since the arterial switch operation includes the transfer of the coronary arteries along with the aortic root, it is important that the surgeon knows exactly what the anatomy is. There are at least nine anatomic variations in the way the two coronary arteries arise from the native aorta. Some coronary patterns are more difficult to transfer than others. In 60% of cases, the coronary arteries come from their appropriate sinuses and branch normally. However, the presence of a ventricular septal defect or side-by-side great vessels should alert the cardiologist to an increased likelihood of coronary anomalies, like left circumflex coronary artery arising from the right coronary artery, or inversion of the coronary arteries origin [18,23].

2.4.2. *Tetralogy of Fallot*

In this disease, the surgical repair includes patch-closure of the ventricular septal defect and widening of the right ventricular outflow tract by infundibular muscle resection combined with either a patch placement across the pulmonary valve annulus or use of a prosthetic conduit from the right ventricle to the pulmonary artery. There are some aberrant coronary patterns associated with tetralogy of Fallot. In some cases, there may be a large conus branch or an accessory left anterior descendent artery running across the face of the right ventricular outflow tract that may be inadvertently damaged during surgery, leading to myocardial ischemia [23].

2.5. Cardiopulmonary bypass and myocardial protection

Recent advances in surgical techniques, myocardial preservation and postoperative care have resulted in complete repair of many CxHD in the neonatal period or early infancy. On the other hand, several investigators have reported that immature myocardium in the paediatric heart is more vulnerable to surgically-induced injury than mature myocardium in the adult heart, due to different structural and functional characteristics [26].

It is widely accepted that the immature heart has a greater tolerance to ischemia than the adult or mature heart. However, most of this laboratory data has been obtained with normal hearts. It is unclear what the ischemic tolerance is when there are pre-existing conditions such as cyanosis, hypertrophy, or acidosis. Many of these conditions may be present in neonates and infants who require surgical correction of their heart defect and may compromise myocardial protection [26].

Newer surgical techniques are being developed to allow for total correction of many CxHD, while limiting the time spent on continuous CPB or in deep hypothermia with circulatory arrest [27]. Therefore, surgeries have been the choice of management in these patients. However, there is a significant procedural- and anaesthesia-related morbidity and mortality in patients with CxHD who undergo repeated surgical interventions [28,29].

Despite of the potentially detrimental side effects of CPB, this technique is still an essential assisting method for open-heart surgery [30]. CPB is a primary circulatory support technique to cardiac surgery in neonates and infants and remains one of the most important factors associated with postoperative mortality and morbidity in open-heart surgery. With improvements in equipment and techniques, CPB has become safer and more reliable. However, it causes profound alterations in physiological fluid homeostasis [31]. The age and size of the patient, the underlying cardiac pathology, and the type of surgical techniques influence what perfusion methods are chosen and the construction of the CPB circuit [32]. Despite significant improvements, CPB remains a non-physiological procedure. The effects of hypothermia, altered perfusion, hemodilution, acid-base management, embolization, and the systemic inflammatory response have been challenging, particularly for neonates and infants. These challenges are primarily related to the smaller circulatory volume, the immaturity of most organ systems, and the increased capillary membrane permeability of neonates and infants [32,33]. Moreover, cardiomyocytes can be affected by hypoxic conditions, and the ischemic effects can induce rapid or gradual changes in the membrane systems that cause reversible or irreversible injury [34]. Experimental studies of myocardial ischemia and reperfusion have established that reperfusion also has negative consequences during circulatory interruption [35,36]. Due to the necessary interruption in coronary circulation required by nearly all cardiac surgeries, the potential for reperfusion damage is significant. If a reperfusion injury does occur, the initial damage may contribute to the impaired cardiac performance that develops immediately after surgery that may then lead to myocardial fibrosis [37,38].

Myocardial preservation during surgically induced myocardial ischemia has been the subject of hundreds of publications in recent years. The most used technique is hypothermic cardioplegia. The consequences of incomplete myocardial protection during surgically induced myocardial ischemia can have a dominant effect on the postoperative course, including low cardiac output, elevated atrial filling pressures, and requirements for increased inotropic support [39]. Cardioplegic solutions are used by most surgeons, and their basic components are potassium (to achieve diastolic arrest) and cold temperature (to reduce the metabolic demands of the heart during ischemia) [39]. There is a variety of different cardioplegic solutions, and there is no consensus on which one is the best. In fact, there is wide variation between institutions regarding cardioplegia and myocardial protection.

Aortic cross clamping during CPB allows the surgeon to intervene on the aortic root, the aortic valve, and the left ventricle outflow tract. However, since during CPB myocardial perfusion is retrograde, during cross clamping the heart is stopped and is not perfused [26,31,39]. Therefore, long cross clamping times are more likely to cause more ischemic injury to the heart.

2.6. Postoperative care and drugs

After surgery, the first 9–12 hours are crucial because during this time the patient will experience a transient decrease in myocardial performance and cardiac output, with increasing need of inotropic support as a consequence of CPB and ischemia-reperfusion injury in the heart and lungs [40]. Besides, the child may deteriorate as a result of residual lesions, pulmonary hypertension, and bleeding. All these factors may lead to poor organ perfusion and hypotension, with consequent reduced coronary blood flow.

In some cases, when the surgical technique involves coronary reimplantation, like the arterial switch for d-TGA, there is a considerable risk of myocardial ischemia. The implantation of the coronary arteries on the neoaorta may be technically challenging, and the coronary insertion may be stenotic or distorted, resulting in insufficient coronary flow. Other causes of insufficient coronary blood flow include spasms of the coronary arteries, air embolism, and thrombosis. Arrhythmias, especially on weaning from CPB, frequently indicate coronary insufficiency; the coronary anastomoses should be promptly investigated before leaving the operating room, as well as transesophageal assessment of left ventricle wall motion. Left ventricular dysfunction may also indicate coronary insufficiency [17].

Many drugs used to improve myocardial contractility and cardiac output can substantially increase myocardial oxygen requirements. In face of hypotension, low cardiac output, or marginally sufficient coronary blood flow, these drugs may actually lead to or aggravate myocardial ischemia. These drugs include dopamine, dobutamine, epinephrine, and norepinephrine.

Arrhythmias, particularly tachyarrhythmias, can also significantly augment the oxygen demand within the myocardium, while compromising the cardiac output, ultimately leading to myocardial ischemia.

Severe blood loss can cause hypotension and a reduction on the arterial oxygen content, substantially affecting oxygen transport to the myocardium.

3. Diagnostic evaluation

3.1. Acute ischemia

Chest pain is the hallmark of myocardial ischemia in adults and the elderly. In children and adolescents, however, the great majority of chest pain episodes are of non-cardiac origin [23]. When myocardial ischemia is present in a critically ill patient admitted to an intensive care unit, there may be no specific sign or symptom, and the diagnosis usually need to be made based on ECG findings and biomarkers alone.

3.1.1. Electrocardiogram

The electrocardiogram (ECG) remains the most important diagnostic test in the evaluation for myocardial ischemia. Many factors are involved in the interpretation if the ECG: age, autonomic tone, heart rate, race, gender, and body habitus. Interestingly, pseudo-abnormal ECGs were found in up to 40% of Olympic athletes with structurally normal hearts [13]. It is important to notice that the ECG should be obtained during the episode or shortly after the event whenever possible; otherwise, the alterations in ECG may disappear. The main ECG findings of myocardial ischemia are ST changes, namely elevation or depression of the ST segment. Although repolarization changes, pericardial diseases, drugs, and electrolyte abnormalities can also cause ST changes, a negative ECG is extremely predictive of non-ischemic events [13].

3.1.2. Biomarkers

When myocardial ischemia occurs, some enzymes from the myocardium are released and can be detected in peripheral blood approximately 2 hours later. The main biomarkers available are cardiac troponins (both I and T) and creatine kinase MD isoenzyme (CK-MB). When elevated, they can diagnose myocardial ischemia with good sensitivity and specificity [13].

3.1.3. Echocardiogram

Echocardiography is the predominant imaging modality used for the diagnosis and management of CxHD because of its widespread availability, ease of use, real-time imaging and cost effectiveness. The role of echocardiography specifically for the detection of myocardial ischemia in the CxHD population is less well established. Furthermore, the indications and clinical applications of other newer echo techniques such as tissue Doppler imaging, strain and strain rate imaging, contrast and real-time three-dimensional (3D) echocardiography to detect myocardial ischemia will need to be determined in these patients [2]. It can be helpful to detect the following: hypertrophic cardiomyopathy, severe aortic stenosis, and dilated cardiomyopathy, all of them potentially associated with coronary flow abnormalities and myocardial ischemia. In some cases, it can show clues to the suspicion of ALCAPA and other coronary abnormalities [13].

3.2. Chronic ischemia

The diagnosis of chronic ischemia in patients with CxHD may be challenging for the physician because this population, often adults operated on early in life, may have pre-existing anatomic, functional, or electrocardiographic abnormalities. They may also have pre-existing coronary disease that, in association with other environmental, metabolic and genetic factors, may increase the risk of coronary insufficiency. However, discussing the diagnosis of these abnormalities is beyond the scope of this chapter.

4. Alterations observed within the myocardium

Myocardial infarction is defined by pathology as myocardial cell death due to prolonged ischemia. Cell death is categorized pathologically by coagulation necrosis and/or contraction band necrosis, which usually evolves through oncosis, but can result to a lesser degree from apoptosis. Mallory, et al, 1939, and Lodge-Patch, 1951 described myocardial infarction as a form of coagulation necrosis in which cells transform into eosinophilic hyaline masses [41,42]. Other types of necrosis are also quite common in myocardial infarction. The term contraction band necrosis [43] have been used to describe degenerative changes of myocardial fibers characterized by a hypercontraction or spasm of the fibers, with the formation of irregular abnormal transverse bands due to compression of adjacent sarcomeres. These changes have been observed in association with electric shock, deficiency of potassium, administration of catecholamines, coronary arterial reperfusion, and death after cardiac surgery [44,45]. Although the primary event leading to the formation of "contraction bands" is unknown, most often they probably develop in areas of reflow [46] or "twilight blood flow" after ischemia [47].

Colliquative myocytolysis, have been used to describe focal lesions, mainly in the subendocardium and in perivascular regions, which were characterized by progressive vacuolization of fibers with lysis of contractile elements until only empty sarcolemmal tubes remain [48]. Schlesinger and Reiner, 1955 have proposed that focal myocytolysis is a result of metabolic imbalances secondary to a large variety of disorders. In contraction band necrosis and colliquative myocytolysis, healing is thought to occur by fibroblastic proliferation, without the usual sequence of changes that occurs with coagulation necrosis. Careful analysis of histologic sections by an experienced observer is necessary to distinguish these entities [49] (Fig. 1).

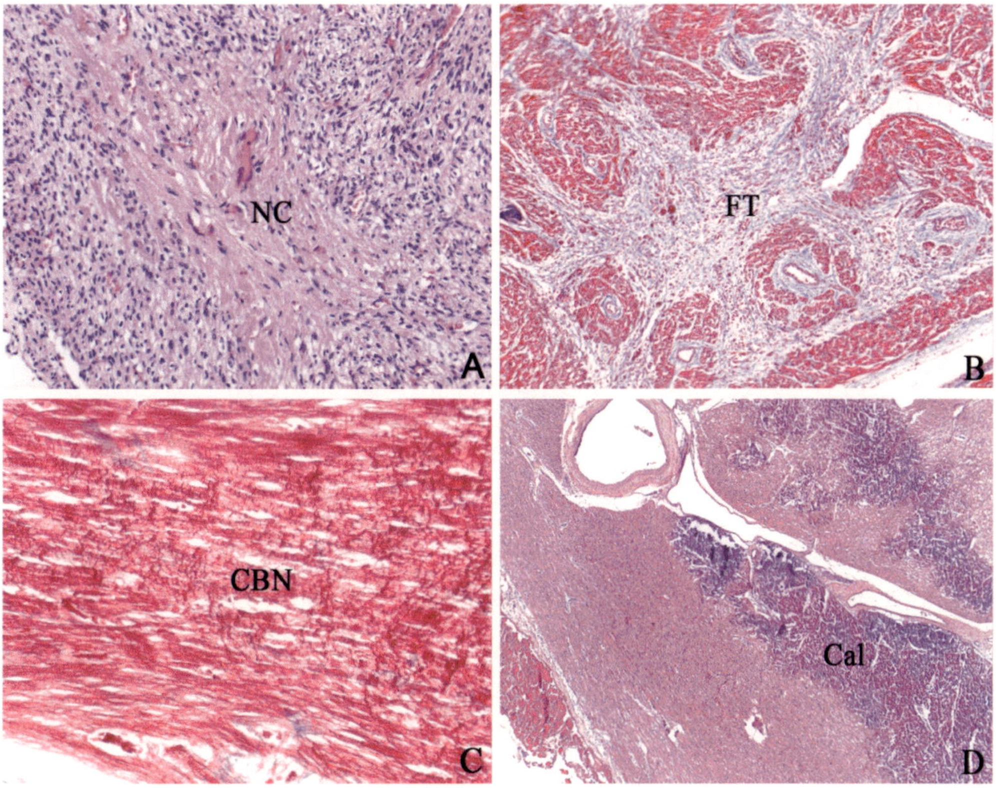

Figure 1. Myocardial injuries observed in infants submitted to cardiac surgery with cardiopulmonary bypass. The histopathology of myocardial injuries observed in infants with congenital cardiac heart disease submitted to surgery with cardiopulmonary bypass (CPB). **(A)** Area of coagulation necrosis (CN) characterized by cells with a cytoplasm that exhibits an increased eosinophilia, loss of cross-striations, granularity, and nuclear karyolysis or pyknosis, H&E; 200x. **(B)** Extensive area of fibrous tissue, Azan; 100x. **(C)** Contraction band necrosis (CBN), Azan; 400x. **(D)** Large calcified intramural band in the myocardium, H&E; 50x.

4.1. Cardiac surgery and myocardial injury

Myocardial injury in association with cardiac surgery can be caused by different mechanisms, including direct trauma by sewing needles, focal trauma from surgical manipulation of the heart, global ischemia from inadequate perfusion, myocardial cell protection or anoxia, and other complications of the procedure [49]. Cardiac surgery with CPB is frequently associated with postoperative organ dysfunction [50]. Paediatric patients are particularly prone to these complications, and oxidative stress seems to contribute to CPB related postoperative complications. Early systemic oxidative stress could also have been a consequence of ischemia-reperfusion injury to the myocardium [51]. It is recognized that acute stress episodes can induce heart injury that results in the release of cytosolic enzymes and catecholamines to the blood [52,53]. Although catecholamines play an important role in normal cardiac function [54], the use of CPB in cardiac surgery leads to a significant increase in circulating catecholamine levels [55,56] and this excessive release is responsible for the development of various cardiac dysfunctions, e.g. in cardiac remodelling following acute myocardial infarction [54], myocyte death in heart failure [57,58], and myocardial infarction [59]. In a recent study, Oliveira, et al, 2011 described that multifocal areas of myocardial injury seem to be the cause of heart failure for infants who do not survive beyond the perioperative period [60]. They were described in patients submitted to surgery for CxHD with and without CPB, and in patients who died from CxHD prior to surgical intervention. Most of the infants who had undergone surgery with CPB showed important areas of contraction band necrosis and dystrophic calcification. Whereas infants who had undergone surgery without CPB showed coagulation necrosis and healing, suggesting ischemia as the main cause. Importantly, 4-hydroxinonenal (4-HNE), a marker of lipid peroxidation, was strongly expressed, especially in irreversible myocardial lesions. This finding suggests that 4-HNE may be the predominant oxidative stress mechanism that occurs in these patients.

4.2. Adrenergic receptors and cardiopulmonary bypass

CPB and cardioplegic arrest remain the most popular techniques in clinical intervention during open-heart surgery. However, both can directly or indirectly result in cardiac morbidity following surgery [61]. Cardioplegic arrest renders the heart globally ischemic and, upon reperfusion, triggers myocardial injury [62]. The use of CPB and cardioplegic arrest during cardiac surgery also leads to desensitization of myocardial β-adrenergic receptors (β-ARs) and impaired signalling through this pathway, which is critical in the regulation of cardiac function [63,64]. Previous studies have demonstrated that cardiac β-AR signalling is impaired after CPB with cardioplegic arrest in children with acyanotic heart disease who underwent cardiac surgery [56]. Adrenergic receptors (ARs), first described by Ahlquist, 1948, belong to the superfamily of membrane proteins that activate heterotrimeric guanine nucleotide (G) binding proteins [65]. The heart expresses both β and $\alpha 1$ adrenergic receptors [66]. The effect of β-adrenergic receptor activation is well established: the increase of both heart rate and force of contraction. The effect of $\alpha 1$-receptor activation is more complex. It is usually described as a biphasic or a triphasic effect: initial positive inotropy, followed by a transient negative and finally a more sustained positive inotropy without effect on chronotropy [67]. In the heart, agonist occupancy of β-ARs leads to the primary activation of the adenylyl cyclase (AC) stimulatory G protein (Gs), which leads to increases in intracellular cAMP and protein kinase A (PKA) activity [68]. Alterations in adrenergic signalling are important in a number of cardiac diseases. Undoubtedly, the alterations that take place in the β-AR system during the progression of heart failure (HF) are the most well characterized [68].

A primary mechanism of β-AR desensitization following prolonged stimulation is phosphorylation of agonist-occupied receptors by G protein-coupled receptor kinase-2 (GRK2), a member of the family of serine-threonine kinases known as G protein-coupled receptor kinases [69]. GRK2 has been shown to be important in the modulation of cardiac function in vivo [70, 71] and enhanced activity leads to uncoupling of β-ARs and impaired ventricular systolic and diastolic function.

Bulcao, et al, 2008 also found significant uncoupling of β-ARs from adenylyl cyclase under basal conditions and following β-agonist stimulation in a patient population following CPB and arrest [72].

In animal studies, inhibition of GRK2 has led to improved myocardial function after ischemic injury [73]. Myocardial GRK2 activity is known to be elevated in patients with chronic heart failure by approximately 2-3-fold compared to normal controls leading to impaired signalling through β-ARs and blunted inotropic reserve [74]. This is thought to be an important mechanism in the pathogenesis of chronic heart failure resulting from an increase in circulating catecholamines [75].During myocardial ischemia, there is a decrease in the supply of oxygen and nutrients to the heart [62]. This, in turn, provokes a fall in energy production by the mitochondria, which is quickly followed by abnormal accumulation and depletion of several intracellular metabolites (e.g. a fall in adenosine triphosphate (ATP) and a rise in lactate). These metabolic changes lead to a decrease in intracellular pH and an increase in the intracellular concentrations of sodium and Ca^{2+}, which further consumes ATP [76], moreover, a local metabolic release of large amounts of noradrenaline occurs [77,78] together with an increased density of β-adrenergic receptors [79-81]. Consecutively, the capacity of β-adrenergic agonists to stimulate adenylate cyclase activity is enhanced during the first 15 minutes of ischemia [79].

With progressive ischemia, however, isoproterenol-stimulated activity of adenylate cyclase decreases to below the control value, although the density of β-receptors remains elevated [80]. This dissociation of receptor number and functional activity has been found in different models of cardiac ischemia [81], including the isolated perfused rat heart [79], and in human myocardium subjected to hypoxia during cardiopulmonary bypass surgery [56].

Similarly, heart failure in humans has also been characterized by specific alterations in the AR signalling system [82]. The enhanced desensitization of myocardial ARs is likely due, at least in part, to the elevated expression of GRK-2 present in human failing heart [74,83]. Mouse models of severe heart failure have been used to demonstrate that inhibition of GRK-2 with a peptide inhibitor can prevent agonist-stimulated desensitization of cardiac β-ARs. This is sufficient to increase mean survival, reduce dilation, and improve cardiac function. This may represent a novel strategy to improve myocardial function in the setting of compromised heart function [70].

5. Strategies for prevention

Prevention of myocardial ischemia in the setting of CxHD is an enormous task. Given the complex pathophysiology, it is very unlikely that a single intervention will show significant reductions on the incidence of myocardial ischemia in patients with CxHD. We can, though, comment on a few of issues that have been matter of investigation recently.

5.1. Before birth

The rate of CxHD that are diagnosed before birth is still low, especially in developing countries, where foetal echocardiography is not widely available. Babies with a prenatal diagnostic of

CxHD may benefit from catheter-based interventions such as balloon valve dilations or device-closure of abnormal communications. These interventions may lead to better intra-uterus myocardial perfusion and development.

5.2. After birth

Babies with CxHD should ideally be delivered in a tertiary-care hospital with a dedicated cardiac paediatric intensive care unit. However, this can only be accomplished by increasing prenatal diagnostic of CxHD, which is known to be limited. Babies with a prenatal diagnostic of CxHD that are delivered in an adequate setting are more likely to receive high quality care and less likely to develop hemodynamic instability and myocardial ischemia.

In addition, a precise anatomic diagnosis is mandatory for an adequate preoperative management, and can help clinical decision making on drugs and dosing, oxygen supplementation, and need for mechanical ventilation.

5.3. During surgery

Only a few episodes of myocardial ischemia occurring during surgical procedures can be attributed to the procedure itself. When the procedures involve repositioning of the coronary arteries, special attention should be put on the technique, but other factors may be equally important. Minimizing the duration of CPB and aortic cross clamping can also help reducing periods of myocardial ischemia. In particular, the type of cardioplegia and myocardial protection may substantially affect the likelihood of ischemia both during and after surgery. Some authors defend that blood cardioplegia may be superior to crystalloid cardioplegia especially for longer (> 1 hour) myocardial ischemic time [26]. However, the superiority of one type of cardioplegic solution over the others is still matter of debate.

5.4. Postoperatively

Immediately after surgery and within the first 24–48 hours, some strategies may significantly reduce the risk of myocardial ischemia following heart surgery, such as: (a) use of coronary vasodilators, like nitroglycerin, especially when the coronary arteries were surgically repositioned; (b) avoiding hypotension; (c) avoiding hyperthermia; (d) minimizing the use of drugs that increase myocardial oxygen demand; (e) keeping the haemoglobin content in blood of at least 10 g/dL; and (f) avoiding tachycardia and aggressively treating tachyarrhythmias. In the setting of hyperthermia, tachyarrhythmias, or low cardiac output syndrome, a mild hypothermia may result in lower oxygen requirements and lower heart rates with better diastolic filling and improved cardiac output.

5.5. Long-term follow-up

Preventive measures for coronary disease in the long term in patients with CxHD are not different from the general population. Dyslipidaemias, chronic arterial hypertension, diet, exercise, are diabetes, among others, shall be managed accordingly. Screening for coronary disease and myocardial ischemia should probably be more frequent and comprehensive in people with CxHD but, to date, there is no additional recommendation for these people in order to prevent coronary disease in the adulthood.

6. Future research

Results of paediatric heart surgery have improved through evolution of surgical techniques, CPB, and paediatric cardiac intensive care over the last several years. These efforts are the result of the collaboration of all subspecialties involved in the care of paediatric patients with CxHD. Despite these advances, the field of paediatric cardiac intensive care is still an exciting, demanding, and evolving discipline, necessitating the ongoing commitment of various disciplines to pursue a greater understanding of disease processes and how to best go about treating them [84].

However, it is very important detect and evaluate the degree of myocardial injury as soon as possible after the operative procedure, in an attempt to clarify possible mechanisms involved in the development of ischemic heart disease in children with CxHD, aiming to discuss potential strategies of the prevent this disease [85].

Future research should focus on molecular mechanisms of myocardial injury, including ischemia-reperfusion injury and the systemic inflammatory response. Clinical trials comparing different myocardial protection strategies and anti-inflammatory drugs are strongly needed. In addition, individualized care based on genetic profiles and the presence of polymorphisms may also contribute to better outcomes.

7. Conclusions

In conclusion, myocardial ischemia following paediatric heart surgery for CxHD is an important issue, probably under diagnosed by physicians, which can lead to catastrophic consequences shortly after surgery or in the long term. The number of people with CxHD reaching adulthood is increasing, and knowing the number of patients with CxHD who were born, who are still alive, and who are reaching adulthood at any given time is required for the adequate allocation of care. These patients are at an increased risk of chronic coronary artery disease and myocardial ischemia. A better understanding of the underlying pathophysiology and the development of screening tests and prophylactic and therapeutic interventions deserve special attention from physicians and researchers.

Acknowledgements

This work was supported by grants from the Fundação de Amparo à Pesquisa do Estado de São Paulo, FAPESP (2010/11.209-0). Simone G. Ramos is a researcher from Conselho Nacional de Desenvolvimento Científico e Tecnológico (CNPq). The authors thank Elaine Medeiros Floriano for technical assistance.

Author details

Fabio Carmona[1*], Karina M. Mata[2], Marcela S. Oliveira[2] and Simone G. Ramos[2]

*Address all correspondence to: carmona@fmrp.usp.br

1 Department of Paediatrics, Faculty of Medicine of Ribeirao Preto, Ribeirao Preto, University of Sao Paulo, Brazil

2 Department of Pathology, Faculty of Medicine of Ribeirao Preto, Ribeirao Preto, University of Sao Paulo, Brazil

References

[1] Wren, C, & Sullivan, O. JJ. Survival with congenital heart disease and need for follow up in adult life. Heart (2001)., 85(4), 438-443.

[2] Tan, J. L, Loong, C. Y, Anagnostopoulos-tzifa, A, Kilner, P. J, Li, W, & Gatzoulis, M. A. Myocardial Ischemia in Congenital Heart Disease: The Role of Noninvasive Imaging. In: Anagnostopoulos CD, Nihoyannopoulos P, Bax JJ, Wall Evd (eds.) Noninvasive Imaging of Myocardial Ischemia. London: Springer-Verlag; (2006)., 287-305.

[3] Mitchell, S. C, Korones, S. B, & Berendes, H. W. Congenital heart disease in 56,109 births. Incidence and natural history. Circulation (1971)., 43(3), 323-332.

[4] Hoffman, J. I, & Kaplan, S. The incidence of congenital heart disease. Journal of the American College of Cardiology (2002)., 39(12), 1890-1900.

[5] Hoffman, J. I. Incidence of congenital heart disease: I. Postnatal incidence. Pediatric Cardiology (1995)., 16(3), 103-113.

[6] Nora, J, Berg, K, & Nora, A. Cardiovascular Diseases. Genetics, Epidemiology and Prevention. New York: Oxford University Press; (1991).

[7] Nora, J. J, & Nora, A. H. Genetic and environmental factors in the etiology of congenital heart diseases. Southern Medical Journal (1976)., 69(7), 919-926.

[8] Kuciene, R, & Dulskiene, V. Selected environmental risk factors and congenital heart defects. Medicina (2008)., 44(11), 827-832.

[9] Kern, J. H, Hinton, V. J, Nereo, N. E, Hayes, C. J, & Gersony, W. M. Early developmental outcome after the Norwood procedure for hypoplastic left heart syndrome. Pediatrics (1998)., 102(5), 1148-1152.

[10] Pillutla, P, Shetty, K. D, & Foster, E. Mortality associated with adult congenital heart disease: Trends in the US population from 1979 to 2005. American Heart Journal (2009)., 158(5), 874-879.

[11] Sadowski, S. L. Congenital cardiac disease in the newborn infant: past, present, and future. Critical Care Nursing Clinics of North America (2009). vi., 21(1), 37-48.

[12] Hasegawa, T, Yamaguchi, M, Yoshimura, N, & Okita, Y. The dependence of myocardial damage on age and ischemic time in pediatric cardiac surgery. The Journal of Thoracic and Cardiovascular Surgery (2005)., 129(1), 192-198.

[13] Daniels, C. J. Myocardial ischemia. In: Allen HD, Driscoll DJ, Shaddy RE, Feltes TF (eds.) Moss and Adams' Heart Disease in Infants, Children, and Adolescents: Including the Fetus and Young Adults. 7th ed. Philadelphia: Lippincott Williams & Wilkins; (2008)., 1312-1321.

[14] Tchervenkov, C. I, Jacobs, J. P, Bernier, P. L, Stellin, G, Kurosawa, H, Mavroudis, C, Jonas, R. A, Cicek, S. M, Al-halees, Z, Elliott, M. J, Jatene, M. B, Kinsley, R. H, Kreutzer, C, Leon-wyss, J, Liu, J, Maruszewski, B, Nunn, G. R, Ramirez-marroquin, S, Sandoval, N, Sano, S, Sarris, G. E, Sharma, R, Shoeb, A, Spray, T. L, Ungerleider, R. M, Yangni-angate, H, & Ziemer, G. The improvement of care for paediatric and congenital cardiac disease across the World: a challenge for the World Society for Pediatric and Congenital Heart Surgery. Cardiology in the Young (2008). Suppl , 2, 63-69.

[15] Zannini, L, & Borini, I. State of the art of cardiac surgery in patients with congenital heart disease. Journal of Cardiovascular Medicine (2007)., 8(1), 3-6.

[16] Stuart, A. G. Changing lesion demographics of the adult with congenital heart disease: an emerging population with complex needs. Future cardiology (2012)., 8(2), 305-313.

[17] Wernovsky, G, & Jonas, R. A. Other conotruncal lesions- Transposition of the great arteries. In: Chang AC, Hanley FL, Wernovsky G, Wessel DL (eds.) Pediatric Cardiac Intensive Care. 1st ed. Baltimore: Williams & Wilkins; (1998)., 289-300.

[18] Matherne, G. P, & Lim, D. S. Congenital Anomalies of the Coronary Vessels and the Aortic Root. In: Allen HD, Driscoll DJ, Shaddy RE, Feltes TF (eds.) Moss and Adams' Heart Disease in Infants, Children, and Adolescents: Including the Fetus and Young Adults. 7th ed. Philadelphia: Lippincott Williams & Wilkins; (2008)., 702-714.

[19] Patterson, A. J, & Zhang, L. Hypoxia and fetal heart development. Current Molecular Medicine (2010)., 10(7), 653-666.

[20] Matter, M, Abdel-hady, H, Attia, G, Hafez, M, Seliem, W, & Al-arman, M. Myocardial Performance in Asphyxiated Full-Term Infants Assessed by Doppler Tissue Imaging. Pediatric Cardiology (2010)., 31(5), 634-642.

[21] Shastri, A. T, Samarasekara, S, Muniraman, H, & Clarke, P. Cardiac troponin I concentrations in neonates with hypoxic-ischaemic encephalopathy. Acta Paediatrica (2011)., 101(1), 26-29.

[22] Keane, J. F, & Fyler, D. C. Coronary artery anomalies. In: Keane JF, Lock JE, Fyler DC (eds.) Nadas' Pediatric Cardiology. Philadelphia: Saunders Elsevier; (2006)., 805-810.

[23] Takahashi, M. Cardiac Ischemia in Pediatric Patients. Pediatric Clinics of North America (2010)., 57(6), 1261-1280.

[24] Hornung, T. S, Kilner, P. J, Davlouros, P. A, Grothues, F, Li, W, & Gatzoulis, M. A. Excessive right ventricular hypertrophic response in adults with the mustard procedure for transposition of the great arteries. The American Journal of Cardiology (2002)., 90(7), 800-803.

[25] Millane, T, Bernard, E. J, Jaeggi, E, Howman-giles, R. B, Uren, R. F, Cartmill, T. B, Hawker, R. E, & Celermajer, D. S. Role of ischemia and infarction in late right ventricular dysfunction after atrial repair of transposition of the great arteries. Journal of the American College of Cardiology (2000)., 35(6), 1661-1668.

[26] Jaggers, J, & Ungerleider, R. M. Cardiopulmonary bypass in infants and children. In: Nichols DG, Ungerleider RM, Spevak PJ, Greeley WJ, Cameron DE, Lappe DG, Wetzel RC (eds.) Critical Heart Disease in Infants and Children. 2nd ed. Philadelphia: Mosby Elsevier; (2006)., 507-528.

[27] Onuzo, O. C. How effectively can clinical examination pick up congenital heart disease at birth? Archives of Disease in Childhood Fetal and Neonatal Edition (2006). F, 236-237.

[28] Giamberti, A, Chessa, M, Abella, R, Butera, G, Carlucci, C, Nuri, H, Frigiola, A, & Ranucci, M. Morbidity and mortality risk factors in adults with congenital heart disease undergoing cardiac reoperations. The Annals of Thoracic Surgery (2009). , 88(4), 1284-1289.

[29] Odegard, K. C. DiNardo JA, Kussman BD, Shukla A, Harrington J, Casta A, McGowan FX, Jr., Hickey PR, Bacha EA, Thiagarajan RR, Laussen PC. The frequency of anesthesia-related cardiac arrests in patients with congenital heart disease undergoing cardiac surgery. Anesthesia and Analgesia (2007)., 105(2), 335-343.

[30] Wang, S, Lv, S, Guan, Y, Gao, G, Li, J, Hei, F, & Long, C. Cardiopulmonary bypass techniques and clinical outcomes in Beijing Fuwai Hospital: a brief clinical review. ASAIO journal (2011)., 57(5), 414-420.

[31] Hirleman, E, & Larson, D. F. Cardiopulmonary bypass and edema: physiology and pathophysiology. Perfusion (2008)., 23(6), 311-322.

[32] Jones, T. J, & Elliott, M. J. Paediatric CPB: bypass in a high risk group. Perfusion (2006)., 21(4), 229-233.

[33] Jonas, R. A, Wypij, D, Roth, S. J, Bellinger, D. C, & Visconti, K. J. du Plessis AJ, Goodkin H, Laussen PC, Farrell DM, Bartlett J, McGrath E, Rappaport LJ, Bacha EA, Forbess JM, del Nido PJ, Mayer JE, Jr., Newburger JW. The influence of hemodilution on outcome after hypothermic cardiopulmonary bypass: results of a randomized trial in infants. The Journal of Thoracic and Cardiovascular Surgery (2003)., 126(6), 1765-1774.

[34] Asano, G, Takashi, E, Ishiwata, T, Onda, M, Yokoyama, M, Naito, Z, Ashraf, M, & Sugisaki, Y. Pathogenesis and protection of ischemia and reperfusion injury in myocardium. Journal of Nihon Medical School (2003). , 70(5), 384-392.

[35] Follette, D. M, Fey, K, Buckberg, G. D, & Helly, J. J. Jr., Steed DL, Foglia RP, Maloney JV, Jr. Reducing postischemic damage by temporary modification of reperfusate calcium, potassium, pH, and osmolarity. The Journal of Thoracic and Cardiovascular Surgery (1981). , 82(2), 221-238.

[36] Buckberg, G. D, & Allen, B. S. Myocardial protection management during adult cardiac operations. In: Baue AE, Geha AS, Hammond GL, Laks H, Naunheim KS (eds.) Glenn's Thoracic and Cardiovascular Surgery. Stamford: Appleton and Lange; (1995). , 1653-1687.

[37] Castañeda, A. R, & Jonas, R. A. Mayer JEJ, Hanley FL. Myocardial preservation in the immature heart. In: Castañeda AR, Jonas RA, Mayer JEJ, Hanley FL (eds.) Cardiac Surgery of the Neonate and Infant. Philadelphia: WB Saunders; (1994). , 41-54.

[38] Kirklin, J, & Barratt-boyes, B. Myocardial management during cardiac surgery with cardiopulmonary bypass. In: Kirklin J, Barrett-Boyes B (eds.) Cardiac Surgery. New York: Churchill Livingstone; (1993). , 129-166.

[39] Mayer Jr JECardiopulmonary bypass. In: Chang AC, Hanley FL, Wernovsky G, Wessel DL (eds.) Pediatric Cardiac Intensive Care. 1st ed. Baltimore: Williams & Wilkins; (1998). , 189-200.

[40] Wernovsky, G, Wypij, D, Jonas, R. A, & Mayer, J. E. Jr., Hanley FL, Hickey PR, Walsh AZ, Chang AC, Castaneda AR, Newburger JW. Postoperative course and hemodynamic profile after the arterial switch operation in neonates and infants. A comparison of low-flow cardiopulmonary bypass and circulatory arrest. Circulation (1995). , 92(8), 2226-2235.

[41] Lodge-patch, I. The ageing of cardiac infarcts, and its influence on cardiac rupture. British Heart Journal (1951). , 13(1), 37-42.

[42] Mallory, G. K, White, P. D, & Salcedo-salgar, J. The speed of healing of myocardial infarcts: A study of the pathologic anatomy in 72 cases. American Heart Journal (1939).

[43] Baroldi, G. Different types of myocardial necrosis in coronary heart disease: a pathophysiologic review of their functional significance. American Heart Journal (1975). , 89(6), 742-752.

[44] Morales, A. R, Fine, G, & Taber, R. E. Cardiac surgery and myocardial necrosis. Archives of Pathology (1967). , 83(1), 71-79.

[45] Reichenbach, D. D, & Benditt, E. P. Myofibrillar degeneration. A response of the myocardial cell to injury. Archives of Pathology (1968). , 85(2), 189-199.

[46] Kloner, R. A, Ganote, C. E, & Whalen, D. A. Jr., Jennings RB. Effect of a transient period of ischemia on myocardial cells. II. Fine structure during the first few minutes of reflow. The American Journal of Pathology (1974). , 74(3), 399-422.

[47] Bouchardy, B, & Majno, G. Histopathology of early myocardial infarcts. A new approach. The American Journal of Pathology (1974). , 74(2), 301-330.

[48] Schlesinger, M. J, & Reiner, L. Focal myocytolysis of the heart. The American Journal of Pathology (1955). , 31(3), 443-459.

[49] Alpert, J. S, Thygesen, K, Antman, E, & Bassand, J. P. Myocardial infarction redefined--a consensus document of The Joint European Society of Cardiology/American College of Cardiology Committee for the redefinition of myocardial infarction. Journal of the American College of Cardiology (2000). , 36(3), 959-969.

[50] Laffey, J. G, Boylan, J. F, & Cheng, D. C. The systemic inflammatory response to cardiac surgery: implications for the anesthesiologist. Anesthesiology (2002). , 97(1), 215-252.

[51] Ferrari, R, Alfieri, O, Curello, S, Ceconi, C, Cargnoni, A, Marzollo, P, Pardini, A, Caradonna, E, & Visioli, O. Occurrence of oxidative stress during reperfusion of the human heart. Circulation (1990). , 81(1), 201-211.

[52] Arakawa, H, Kodama, H, Matsuoka, N, & Yamaguchi, I. Stress increases plasma enzyme activity in rats: differential effects of adrenergic and cholinergic blockades. The Journal of Pharmacology and Experimental Therapeutics (1997). , 280(3), 1296-1303.

[53] Meltzer, H. Y. Plasma creatine phosphokinase activity, hypothermia, and stress. The American Journal of Physiology (1971). , 221(3), 896-901.

[54] Piano, M. R, & Prasun, M. Neurohormone activation. Critical Care Nursing Clinics of North America (2003). , 15(4), 413-421.

[55] Minami, K, Korner, M. M, Vyska, K, Kleesiek, K, Knobl, H, & Korfer, R. Effects of pulsatile perfusion on plasma catecholamine levels and hemodynamics during and after cardiac operations with cardiopulmonary bypass. The Journal of Thoracic and Cardiovascular Surgery (1990). , 99(1), 82-91.

[56] Schranz, D, Droege, A, Broede, A, Brodermann, G, Schafer, E, Oelert, H, & Brodde, O. E. Uncoupling of human cardiac beta-adrenoceptors during cardiopulmonary bypass with cardioplegic cardiac arrest. Circulation (1993). , 87(2), 422-426.

[57] Carelock, J, & Clark, A. P. Heart failure: pathophysiologic mechanisms. The American Journal of Nursing (2001). , 101(12), 26-33.

[58] Goldspink, D. F, Burniston, J. G, & Tan, L. B. Cardiomyocyte death and the ageing and failing heart. Experimental Physiology (2003). , 88(3), 447-458.

[59] Ueyama, T, Senba, E, Kasamatsu, K, Hano, T, Yamamoto, K, Nishio, I, Tsuruo, Y, & Yoshida, K. Molecular mechanism of emotional stress-induced and catecholamine-induced heart attack. Journal of Cardiovascular Pharmacology (2003). Suppl 1:S, 115-118.

[60] Oliveira, M. S, Floriano, E. M, Mazin, S. C, Martinez, E. Z, Vicente, W. V, Peres, L. C, Rossi, M. A, & Ramos, S. G. Ischemic myocardial injuries after cardiac malformation repair in infants may be associated with oxidative stress mechanisms. Cardiovascular Pathology (2011). e, 43-52.

[61] Suleiman, M. S, Zacharowski, K, & Angelini, G. D. Inflammatory response and cardioprotection during open-heart surgery: the importance of anaesthetics. British Journal of Pharmacology (2008). , 153(1), 21-33.

[62] Suleiman, M. S, Halestrap, A. P, & Griffiths, E. J. Mitochondria: a target for myocardial protection. Pharmacology & Therapeutics (2001). , 89(1), 29-46.

[63] Booth, J. V, Landolfo, K. P, Chesnut, L. C, Bennett-guerrero, E, Gerhardt, M. A, Atwell, D. M, Moalem, H. E, Smith, M. S, Funk, B. L, Kuhn, C. M, Kwatra, M. M, & Schwinn, D. A. Acute depression of myocardial beta-adrenergic receptor signaling during cardiopulmonary bypass: impairment of the adenylyl cyclase moiety. Duke Heart Center Perioperative Desensitization Group. Anesthesiology (1998). , 89(3), 602-611.

[64] Schwinn, D. A, Leone, B. J, Spahn, D. R, Chesnut, L. C, Page, S. O, Mcrae, R. L, & Liggett, S. B. Desensitization of myocardial beta-adrenergic receptors during cardiopulmonary bypass. Evidence for early uncoupling and late downregulation. Circulation (1991). , 84(6), 2559-2567.

[65] Caron, M. G, & Lefkowitz, R. J. Catecholamine receptors: structure, function, and regulation. Recent Progress in Hormone Research (1993). , 48, 277-290.

[66] Brodde, O. E, & Michel, M. C. Adrenergic and muscarinic receptors in the human heart. Pharmacological Reviews (1999). , 51(4), 651-690.

[67] Terzic, A, Puceat, M, Vassort, G, & Vogel, S. M. Cardiac alpha 1-adrenoceptors: an overview. Pharmacological Reviews (1993). , 45(2), 147-175.

[68] Brodde, O. E. Beta-adrenoceptors in cardiac disease. Pharmacology & Therapeutics (1993). , 60(3), 405-430.

[69] Rockman, H. A, Koch, W. J, & Lefkowitz, R. J. Seven-transmembrane-spanning receptors and heart function. Nature (2002). , 415(6868), 206-212.

[70] Akhter, S. A, Eckhart, A. D, Rockman, H. A, Shotwell, K, Lefkowitz, R. J, & Koch, W. J. In vivo inhibition of elevated myocardial beta-adrenergic receptor kinase activity in hybrid transgenic mice restores normal beta-adrenergic signaling and function. Circulation (1999). , 100(6), 648-653.

[71] Koch, W. J, Rockman, H. A, Samama, P, Hamilton, R. A, Bond, R. A, Milano, C. A, & Lefkowitz, R. J. Cardiac function in mice overexpressing the beta-adrenergic receptor kinase or a beta ARK inhibitor. Science (1995). , 268(5215), 1350-1353.

[72] Bulcao, C. F, Pandalai, P. K, Souza, D, Merrill, K. M, & Akhter, W. H. SA. Uncoupling of myocardial beta-adrenergic receptor signaling during coronary artery bypass grafting: the role of GRK2. The Annals of Thoracic Surgery (2008). , 86(4), 1189-1194.

[73] White, D. C, Hata, J. A, Shah, A. S, Glower, D. D, Lefkowitz, R. J, & Koch, W. J. Preservation of myocardial beta-adrenergic receptor signaling delays the development of heart failure after myocardial infarction. Proceedings of the National Academy of Sciences of the United States of America (2000). , 97(10), 5428-5433.

[74] Ungerer, M, Bohm, M, Elce, J. S, Erdmann, E, & Lohse, M. J. Altered expression of beta-adrenergic receptor kinase and beta 1-adrenergic receptors in the failing human heart. Circulation (1993). , 87(2), 454-463.

[75] Ungerer, M, Kessebohm, K, Kronsbein, K, Lohse, M. J, & Richardt, G. Activation of beta-adrenergic receptor kinase during myocardial ischemia. Circulation Research (1996). , 79(3), 455-460.

[76] Halestrap, A. P. Mitochondria and reperfusion injury of the heart--a holey death but not beyond salvation. Journal of Bioenergetics and Biomembranes (2009). , 41(2), 113-121.

[77] Schomig, A. Catecholamines in myocardial ischemia. Systemic and cardiac release. Circulation (1990). Suppl):II, 13-22.

[78] Schomig, A, Dart, A. M, Dietz, R, Mayer, E, & Kubler, W. Release of endogenous catecholamines in the ischemic myocardium of the rat. Part A: Locally mediated release. Circulation Research (1984). , 55(5), 689-701.

[79] Strasser, R. H, Krimmer, J, Braun-dullaeus, R, Marquetant, R, & Kubler, W. Dual sensitization of the adrenergic system in early myocardial ischemia: independent regulation of the beta-adrenergic receptors and the adenylyl cyclase. Journal of Molecular and Cellular Cardiology (1990). , 22(12), 1405-1423.

[80] Vatner, D. E, Knight, D. R, Shen, Y. T, & Thomas, J. X. Jr., Homcy CJ, Vatner SF. One hour of myocardial ischemia in conscious dogs increases beta-adrenergic receptors, but decreases adenylate cyclase activity. Journal of Molecular and Cellular Cardiology (1988). , 20(1), 75-82.

[81] Vatner, D. E, Young, M. A, Knight, D. R, & Vatner, S. F. Beta-receptors and adenylate cyclase: comparison of nonischemic, ischemic, and postmortem tissue. The American Journal of Physiology (1990). Pt 2):H, 140-144.

[82] Feldman, A. M. Modulation of adrenergic receptors and G-transduction proteins in failing human ventricular myocardium. Circulation (1993). Suppl):IV, 27-34.

[83] Ungerer, M, Parruti, G, Bohm, M, Puzicha, M, Deblasi, A, Erdmann, E, & Lohse, M. J. Expression of beta-arrestins and beta-adrenergic receptor kinases in the failing human heart. Circulation Research (1994). , 74(2), 206-213.

[84] Bronicki, R. A, & Chang, A. C. Management of the postoperative pediatric cardiac surgical patient. Critical Care Medicine (2011). , 39(8), 1974-1984.

http://dx.doi.org/10.5772/53420

[85] Van Der Bom, T, Zomer, A. C, Zwinderman, A. H, Meijboom, F. J, Bouma, B. J, & Mulder, B. J. The changing epidemiology of congenital heart disease. Nature Reviews Cardiology (2011). , 8(1), 50-60.

Chapter 3

Significance of Arterial Endothelial Dysfunction and Possibilities of Its Correction in Silent Myocardial Ischemia and Diabetes Mellitus

I.P. Tatarchenko, N.V. Pozdnyakova, O.I. Morozova,
A.G. Mordovina, S.A. Sekerko and I.A. Petrushin

Additional information is available at the end of the chapter

http://dx.doi.org/10.5772/53445

1. Introduction

The high rate of disability and mortality among patients with Diabetes Mellitus (DM) is mainly caused by cardiovascular disorders. The pathogenic effect of a number of specific factors (hyperglycemia, hyperinsulinemia, insulin resistance) accelerates the development and progression of the diseases connected with atherosclerosis. They are the main causes of death among population of industrialized countries. The incidence of cardiovascular disease is 3-4 times higher among patients with Type II DM in comparison with patients having normal carbohydrate metabolism. However, atypical clinical course of coronary heart disease makes diagnosis of coronary insufficiency among patients with DM rather difficult. It results in later detection of disease, i.e. the disease is often detected on the stage of severe complications such as sudden death or circulatory failure [1]. According to Thomas Killip [2], asymptomatic myocardial ischemia occurs 2-4 times more often in diabetes, while Cohn P.F. and Fox K.M. [3] say about 5-fold increased risk of cardiac mortality among patients with asymptomatic myocardial ischemia. It should be noted that the presence of silent myocardial ischemia increases the risk of complications such as acute myocardial infarction and unstable angina [4].

Although pathogenetic mechanisms of the appearance of silent and pain ischemia are considered to be the same and they are caused by mismatch between myocardial oxygen demand and coronary blood flow we still do not have a clear answer on the question about causes of asymptomatic myocardial ischemia.

The absence of pain among patients with DM is connected with loss of sensitivity of opioid receptors to adenosine which is one of the mediators of cardiac pain [3]. Other researchers believe that the main cause of the development of silent myocardial ischemia is diabetic autonomic neuropathy [5;6]. According to Kempler P. [7], 24-hour monitoring showed that 64.7% patients having DM with diabetic autonomic neuropathy suffered silent ischemia while only 4.1% patients having DM without diabetic autonomic neuropathy suffered silent ischemia.

Undoubtedly, diagnostic methods allowing the detection of disease before the development of dangerous conditions are important in the absence of characteristic clinical symptoms among patients with DM. Early diagnosis of coronary heart disease is particularly necessary.

The role of endothelial dysfunction in the formation of vascular complications attracts attention of clinicians. The vascular endothelium certainly plays a key role in maintaining normal vascular tone and structure, local homeostasis and processes of cell proliferation of the vascular wall [8, 9]. The vascular endothelium is considered to be metabolically active tissue formed by a corporation of specialized cells. It secretes both vasoconstrictors (angiotensin II, endothelin, free radicals of incompletely oxidized fatty acids, prostaglandin F2 alpha, thromboxane) and vasodilators (nitric oxide (NO), endothelial hyperpolarizing factor, prostacyclin), their effects are balanced under physiological conditions. The dysfunction of endothelial cells causes increased vascular permeability for macromolecules [10], changes in the level of vasoactive substances and vascular expansion and vasospasm respectively [11; 12] and change in the balance of coagulation and anticoagulation systems [13]. However, endothelial dysfunction most often leads to changes in the vascular lumen. Endothelial cell dysfunction is considered to be the change in the vascular response to the delivery acetylcholine into the bloodstream and hyperemia which normally lead to vasodilatation due to release of NO.

In DM the ability of endothelial cells to synthesize NO is reduced [14; 15], the ability of endothelial cells to release relaxing factors decreases while the formation of vasoconstrictive factors persists or increases, i.e. the imbalance between the neurotransmitters providing the best rate for all endothelium-dependent processes is formed. This condition is defined as endothelial dysfunction. The major manifestations of endothelial dysfunction are violation of the endothelium relaxation of blood vessels and increased adhesiveness of endothelial lining [16].

As Tooke J. noted, insulin may affect the endothelium of blood vessels in two ways causing them to either expand or spasm [17]. Binding to its receptors on the surface of endothelial cells insulin may act in two ways. The first way is an activation of NO secretion through the insulin receptor substrate 1 and substrate 2 (IRS-1, IRS-2) and phosphatidylinositol-3-kinase (PI3-K). This mechanism provides a vasodilator and antiatherogenic properties of insulin; it is involved in insulin-dependent delivery of glucose into cells. The second way is implementation of the mitogenic properties of insulin through a cascade of mediators (ras, raf, MEK) that increase the activity of mitogen-activated protein kinase, which ends with cell proliferation and migration of smooth muscle cells, activation of vasoconstrictor factor endothelin-1 and increased blood pressure [18]. The first mechanism appeared not to function in conditions of insulin resistance. It was the first way which was resistant to insulin; therefore, NO molecule was not synthesized. At the same time, the second mechanism retains its high activity, so, hyperinsulinemia has atherogenic effects.

http://dx.doi.org/10.5772/53445

Endothelial dysfunction of the coronary arteries manifests in reduced coronary flow reserve, inability of vessels to adequate expansion with an increase in myocardial oxygen demand. It has a significant influence on the occurrence and progression of ischemia. Changes in vascular reactivity have an impact on atherogenesis processes, hyperglycemia provokes the primary foci of atheromatous lesions of the vascular wall and creates the conditions for the formation of specific cellular component atheroma [19]. Violation of endothelial function is believed to be an important independent risk factor for coronary heart disease [20], that is why the correction of endothelial dysfunction and control of traditional risk factors for atherosclerosis should be considered as a strategic line of the effective prevention of cardiovascular complications.

According to Schachinger V. and colleages [21], patients with risk of coronary atherosclerosis traditionally suffer endothelial dysfunction of the coronary vessels, but it functions as a long-term marker of the progression of atherosclerosis and cardiovascular events when coronary heart disease is diagnosed. However, this assumption is not supported by all the researchers. A significant difference in the prevalence of silent myocardial ischemia, depending on the presence of DM is a matter of opinion too.

2. The subject and the methods of the research

Having conducted our research, we investigated the relationship between the severity of silent myocardial ischemia and functional state of arteries endothelium, we studied the significance of violations of vasomotor function with the loss of the ability to flow-dependent vasodilation as a risk factor, which increases the probability of the episodes of silent myocardial ischemia among patients with Type II DM.

To conduct the research we formed a group of patients with stable clinical course of coronary heart disease during the previous month. All patients including people with Type II DM had stable sinus rhythm. The research was conducted on condition that the patients took oral antidiabetic drugs. The elimination criteria were Grade 3 hypertension (blood pressure was above 180/110 mmHg); the presence of valvular heart disease and congestive heart failure 3-4 functional class; the presence of chronic liver and renal failure; chronic lung disease with respiratory failure; a history of cerebral stroke.

We observed 128 patients (66 male and 62 female), average age was 59.3±4.7. Each patient signed an agreement to take part in our research as a volunteer. The agreement was adopted by the local ethics committee.

We included patients with coronary heart disease and Type II DM into group 1 (n=60). Duration of diabetes was 6.4±1.5 years. The level of fasting plasma glucose was 7.7±1.5 mmol/l. Group 2 (n=68) was formed by patients having coronary heart disease without violation of carbohydrate metabolism (table 1).

The complex survey included clinical and laboratory studies, 12-lead electrocardiography, Holter ECG monitoring, stress testing (Bruce R. protocol), echocardiography, and ultrasound vascular assessment of endothelium-dependent vasodilation of the brachial artery (BA).

Rate	Group 1 n= 60	Group 2 n= 68
Male/Female (n)	26 / 34	40 / 28
Age (years)	59.8 ± 4.3	58.7 ± 4.8
Smoking (Male/Female, n)	24 / 5	32 / 4
BMI (kg/м^2)	33.1 ± 3.6	28.7 ± 3.1
Arterial hypertension		
degree (n/%) I	35 / 58.3	20 / 69.7
II	21 / 35	10 / 30.3
Stable angina (n):		
I Functional Class	14	15
II Functional Class	24	28
III Functional Class	22	25
Burdened hereditary history		
DM (n/%)	48 / 80	8 / 11.8
CD (n/%)	52 / 86.7	61 / 89.7
Duration of illness (years)		
coronary heart disease	6.4 ± 1.5	5.9 ± 3.2
arterial hypertension	12.3 ± 3.5	13.4 ± 3.5
diabetes mellitus	8.7 ± 2.2	-
hyper Dyslipidemia (n/%)	54 / 90	53 / 77.9
signs of CHF,%	42 / 60	37 / 54.4

Note: BMI - Body Mass Index; CHF - Chronic Heart Failure; CD - Cardiovascular Disease; hyper Dyslipidemia- total cholesterol is more than 5.0 mmol/l and/or low-density lipoprotein cholesterol is more than 3 mmol/l when high density lipoprotein cholesterol is less than 1 mmol/l; n - the absolute number of individuals with this figure; % - number of persons with this figure from the total number of persons enrolled in the study.

Table 1. Clinical characteristics of patients

Vascular Doppler ultrasound was conducted before 10 a.m. when a patient was fasting. The patient had a 10-minute rest before the test. During the test the patient was lying on his/her back. Having scanned the common carotid artery, the brachial artery, common femoral artery and tibial arteries we used a linear detector with the ability to visualize the image in the frequency range 5-12 Hz.

In B-mode we studied the following parameters: vascular permeability; vascular geometry (the correspondence of vascular duct to the anatomical vessel trajectory); the diameter of the vessel (intraluminal); the condition of the vascular wall (the integrity, the thickness of the intima-media (Figure 1.), echogenicity, the degree of differentiation of the layers, the shape of the surface); the state of the vessel lumen (presence, location, length, echogenicity of intraluminal structures, the degree of obstruction); the state of the perivascular tissue (presence, shape, extent, cause extravasal impact). In spectral Doppler mode, we analyzed quantitative indicators of blood flow: peak systolic blood flow velocity (V_{ps}, cm/s); the maximum end diastolic blood flow velocity (V_{ed}, cm/s); diastolic blood flow velocity (V_{d}, cm/s), evaluated in arteries with high peripheral resistance; maximum blood flow velocity, averaged over time (TAMX, cm/s); peripheral resistance index - RI.

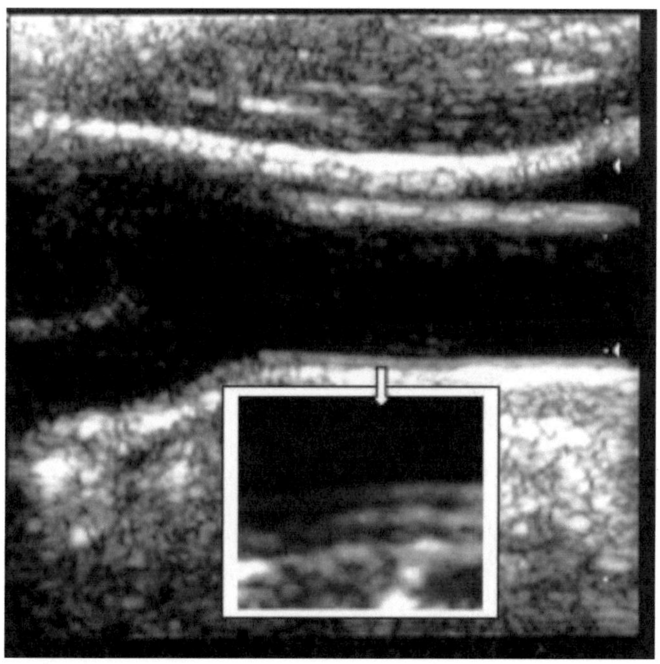

Figure 1. Assessment of intima-media for ultrasound scanning in B-mode

To assess vasomotor function of vascular endothelium, we used a test with reactive hyperemia, i.e. detection of endothelium-dependent vasodilation of the BA by the method of Celermaer D.S. and Sorensen K.E. [22]. The sensor was located in the longitudinal section of a 3 - 4 cm above the elbow. First, the diameter of the BA and the velocity of blood flow through it were measured. Reactive hyperemia was produced by applying a sphygmomanometer cuff on the upper third of the shoulder. During 3-4 minutes we maintained the cuff pressure in this patient greater than systolic pressure by 40 mm Hg. After decompression, the next measurements were carried out in 60 seconds. Endothelium dependent vasodilatation was calculated by the following formula:

Endothelium dependent vasodilatation= ((BA diameter after the test - initial diameter of the BA)/initial diameter of the BA)×100%.

The degree of increase in BA diameter of more than 10% was regarded as a preserved endothelium dependent vasodilatation. In violation of endothelium vasomotor function of BA diameter increase was less than 10%. We got more information on the status of endothelial vasomotor function using the method of transcranial duplex scanning with the stress test, which activates the metabolic mechanisms of influence on the endothelium, i.e. breath holding test. We analyzed the nature of response to the functional stress test, taking into account the index of reactivity:

1. positive - the index of reactivity was from 1.1 to 1.4;
2. negative - the index of reactivity was 0.9 to 1.1;
3. paradoxical - the index of reactivity was less than 0.9 [23].

ECG monitoring was conducted in the ordinary daily routine of a patient. The patient was to keep a diary during ECG recording; he or she recorded the nature of his/her activities and his/her state of health in detail. Besides a computer decoding, the analysis of the results of our research included visual viewing of individual fragments of the ECG recording, which increased the reliability of conclusions. We analyzed ischemic changes, taking into account corrections of the original position in ST segment whether it was ST segment elevation or depression (Figure 2.).

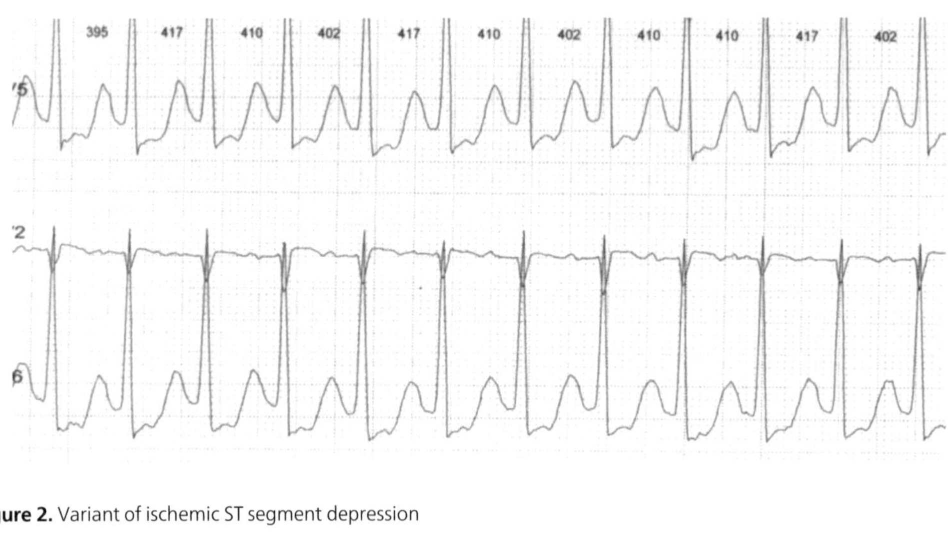

Figure 2. Variant of ischemic ST segment depression

When evaluating each episode, we noted the presence or absence of pain (according to a patient's diary or a marker on the monitor records; we calculated the total duration of daily depression of ST segment (daily myocardial ischemia), a maximum depth of ST segment depression ($\downarrow ST_{max}$), heart rate (HR) at the beginning of painful and painless episodes of ST displacement.

Statistical processing and analysis of the results obtained are presented in the system of statistical analysis STATISTIKA (the package of applied programs STATISTIKA by company StatSoft Inc., Version 6.0.).

3. The results of the research and the discussion

In countries that have achieved significant success in treatment and prevention of coronary heart disease, patients with DM are the only group in which the death rate from this disease has slightly decreased among men and increases among women [24]. In this connection, the data of clinical analysis and comparative evaluation of ischemic episodes based on the results of daily monitoring of ECG and stress testing in groups I and II (Table 2) are of considerable interest.

Rate	Group 1 n=60	Group 2 n=68
The presence of SMI (n)	56 / 93.3%*	40 / 58.8%
Number of painful episode of myocardial ischemia	2.1 ± 0.3	2.1 ± 0.43
Number of silent myocardial ischemia	2.8 ± 0.4*	1.1 ± 0.3
DMI (min)	45.3 ± 3.2*	33.6 ± 2.4
PEMI (min)	14.7 ± 2.5	15.2 ± 1.7
Silent myocardial ischemia (min)	31.1 ± 2.1*	18.6 ± 2.2
The depth of ST segment depression (mm)		
average	1.53 ± 0.4	1.5 ± 0.2
maximum	2.5 ± 0.2*	1.8 ± 0.3
Average heart rate(beats / min)		
at the beginning of PEMI	116 ± 2.3	122 ± 1.8
at the beginning of SMI	97 ± 1.9*	108 ± 3.1
VA during episodes of ischemia (n/%)	12 / 20*	8 / 11.8
The volume of work done (Watt)	400 ± 20*	580 ± 20
The threshold power of load (Watt)	66.5 ± 2.3*	83.3 ± 2.8
Time of occurrence		
ST segment depression (min)	6.7 ± 0.3*	8.6 ± 0.4
Time of pain occurrence (min)	7.3 ± 0.4	8.5 ± 0.7
The number of leads with ST depression	6.3 ± 0.4*	4.4 ± 0.2

Note: DMI - Daily Myocardial Ischemia (duration of ischemic episodes per day); SMI - Silent Myocardial Ischemia; PEMI - Painful Episode of Myocardial Ischemia; VA - Ventricular Arrhythmia; *- $p < 0.05$ – a significant difference.

Table 2. Comparative analysis of functional methods

In group 1 we observed periods of silent ischemia among 93.3% patients, painful episodes of myocardial ischemia were detected in the form of compressive retrosternal pain, discomfort in the chest and dyspnea among 66.7% patients. When analyzing daily trend of ST segment and patients' diary records, we registered a combination of painful episodes of myocardial ischemia and silent myocardial ischemia in 60% cases. Only 6.7% patients with Type II DM had painful episodes of myocardial ischemia while 33.3% patients had ischemic depression episodes of ST segment without any subjective manifestations. That was a significant difference in comparison with the corresponding figures in group 2, χ^2=5.4 ($p<0.05$).

In group 2 episodes of silent myocardial ischemia were detected in 9 (13.2%) cases during a day, the detection rate of painful episodes of myocardial ischemia was 59 (88.6%) cases, 28 (41.2%) patients having had only painful episodes of myocardial ischemia. According to diary records, 51.7% patients with coronary heart disease had a combination of painful episodes of myocardial ischemia and silent myocardial ischemia. A significant difference was obtained by assessing the duration of all episodes of myocardial ischemia during the day in group 1 and group 2, it was 45.3±3.2 min and 33.6±2.4 min< $p<0.03$ accordingly.

The average depth of ST segment depression did not differ significantly among patients of both groups. However, maximum depth of ST depression in group 1 exceeded the same indicator in group 2, it was 2.4±0.2 mm and 1.6±0.3 mm, $p<0.05$ accordingly. The value of heart rate at the beginning of pain and painless episodes did not differ significantly according to groups.

The amount of work done and threshold power were lower among patients of group 1 than patients of group 2. 85% patients of group 1 had ischemic displacement of ST segment, it was detected in more than 6-lead ECG during stress testing.

Measuring the ability to perceive pain which is associated with transient myocardial ischemia has a prognostic value in stable angina. Angina/the equivalent of angina is a signal for patients to regulate their daily physical activity.

We should note that later attack of pain with a delay relatively to the ischemic ST segment shift was detected among 27(45%) patients of group 1 during stress test. In 31 (51.7%) cases the emergence of pain coincided with the appearance of ischemic symptoms on the electrocardiogram. However, in 2 cases the pain occurred before the appearance of ST depression. Having analyzed the results, we obtained different data in group 2: the number of patients with premature/simultaneous appearance of angina/its equivalent was 85.3% and it exceeded the number of patients with late appearance of pain attack (14.7%), $p<0.02$. We assume that data on the detection rate during stress testing of patients with the later occurrence of the attack/equivalent of angina with respect to ischemic ST segment shift (45% and 14.7% - $p<0.03$ respectively), obtained in group 1 in comparison with group 2 may be explained by increased sensitivity to pain among patients with insulin resistant diabetes. It is associated with a change in neuronal component of pain inhibition system, which includes not only the conductors of pain sensitivity, but peripheral receptors in the myocardium.

The data obtained are consistent with the results of daily monitoring of the ECG. The probability of occurrence of asymptomatic episodes of ST depression is significantly higher among patients having coronary heart disease and DM than among patients with coronary heart disease without violation of carbohydrate metabolism. Ratio silent myocardial ischemia/ painful episodes of myocardial ischemia was 1.29 in group 1, and it exceeded the same indicator among patients of group 2 – 0.52 (χ^2=3.84, p<0.05).

However, in our opinion, the pathogenesis of silent myocardial ischemia with violation of carbohydrate metabolism is complex; it appears to be related not only to autonomous cardiac neuropathy, but also to the development of angiopathy, microcirculation disturbance.

It should be noted that the presence and severity of endothelial dysfunction among patients with documented lesions of coronary arteries is a proven marker of poor prognosis [25]. However, this large-scale destruction of the vascular bed does not occur for any other disease, like DM; this is due to the influence of hyperglycemia on the primary target cell, vascular endothelium. Studies carried out in a clinical setting, showed that in DM endothelial dysfunction is associated with microangiopathy and atherosclerosis [26; 27].

When studying functional characteristics of vascular endothelium in the analyzed groups we paid special attention to the results on detecting endothelium-dependent vasodilation of the BA (Table 3).

Rate	Group 1		Group 2	
	initially	after the test	initially	after the test
Diameter of the BA (mm)	3.8 ± 0.19	3.94 ± 0.11**	4.07 ± 0.18	4.57 ± 0.12*
Vps (m/s)	0.62 ± 0.04	0.84 ± 0.06	0.64 ± 0.05	0.92 ± 0.04*
Ved (m/s)	0.10 ± 0.05	0.13 ± 0.03	0.12 ± 0.06	0.16 ± 0.03*
TAMX (m/s)	0.12 ± 0.03	0.29 ± 0.06**	0.13± 0.02	0.43 ± 0.04*
EDV BA (%)	3.7 ± 1.1**		12.3 ± 2.1%	

Note: Vps - Peak systolic blood flow velocity; Ved - maximum end diastolic flow velocity; TAMX - the time-averaged maximum velocity of blood flow; EDV BA - endothelium dependent vasodilation of brachial artery; *- p< 0.05 - reliability of differences between parameters obtained initially and after the test; ** - p< 0.05 - difference is reliable between indicators of group 1 and group 2.

Table 3. Performance test with reactive hyperemia in groups of patients

The original diameter of the BA did not differ significantly in the analyzed groups; it was 3.8±0.19 mm and 4.07±0.18 mm, respectively. Evaluating the mechanism of endothelial regulation of vascular tone among patients in group 1, in the presence of DM, we diagnosed vasomotor endothelial dysfunction induced by shear stress in all cases. The diameter of the BA increased after removal of the cuff by only 3.7±1.1% of the initial indicator in the group. At the same time 53.3% (32) of patients had violation of endothelial vasomotor function as a lack of vasodilating effect, i.e., less than 10% of the original value, 26.7% (16) of patients had violation of endothelial vasomotor function as the lack of increase in BA diameter, and 20%

(12) of patients had violation of endothelial vasomotor function in the form of pathological vasoconstriction.

An interesting fact is that endothelial dysfunction induced by shear stress was detected in the form of lack of increase in BA diameter and pathological vasoconstriction among patients with Type II DM (33.3% of the total number of patients in group 1) having episodes of silent myocardial ischemia without subjective symptoms, it was 15% и 18.3% of cases accordingly.

Correlation analysis showed a significant negative correlation between endothelial dysfunction and the presence of silent myocardial ischemia ($R= -0.68$, $p<0.01$), duration of episodes of silent myocardial ischemia ($R= -0.53$, $p<0.01$), lag time of pain in relation to coronary ST depression ($R= -0.61$, $p<0.01$) in group 1.

We have received reliable dependence of endothelium dependent vasodilation from the functional class (FC) of angina ($R= -0.4215$, $p <0.04$): endothelium dependent vasodilation was 2.4±0.3% in stable angina of FC III, that was significantly less than similar indicator among patients with angina of FC I and FC II, it was 5.2± 0.2% and 4.05±0.15% ($p <0.03$), respectively.

In group 2 index of endothelium dependent vasodilation of BA was 12.3±2.1%. We did not reveal any violations of the vasomotor function of vascular endothelium among 44.1% (30) of patients of this group (endothelium dependent vasodilation was more than 10%). Endothelial dysfunction was registered in 38 (40%) cases: in 29 (42.6%) cases patients suffered lack of growth in BA diameter (endothelium dependent vasodilation was less than 10%), 7 (10.3%) patients had no increase in BA diameter and only 2(3%) patients suffered pathological vasoconstriction.

In Doppler test of linear velocity rates of blood flow of BA (peak systolic blood flow velocity (Vps), maximum end diastolic flow velocity (Ved)), the time-averaged maximum velocity of blood flow (TAMX) did not differ significantly in the groups. However, the degree of increase of the velocity indicators in comparison with reactive hyperemia test was significantly higher in group 2, which also shows a decrease in vasodilating reserve in group 2.

Table 4 presents the results of the analysis of quantitative and qualitative assessment of intima-media complex (IMC) of the arteries of the lower limb arteries, common carotid artery (CCA) and the analysis of cerebrovascular reactivity in these tests with breath-holding.

The thickness of IMC of patients in group 1 was 1.24±0,06 mm in the CCA, in the common femoral artery (CFA) it was 1.32±0.07 mm, the numerical values of these indices were higher than similar indicators among patients of group 2, $p<0.05$. Doing a qualitative analysis of the IMC state we revealed three different types of changes among patients with Type II DM: diffuse uniform thickening of the IMC with the appearance of additional layers of high and low echogenicity in the structure of the intima-media in the CFA, the superficial femoral artery (SFA), the popliteal artery (PA), the posterior tibial artery (PTA), the anterior tibial artery (ATA) (100% patients); in the CCA (95% patients); presence of multiple local zones of increased echogenicity with visualization of atherosclerotic plaques in the structure of IMC (95% were in the PTA and the ATA, 80% were in the PA, 71.7% were in the CFA and SFA; 66.7% patients had it the CCA), increased echogenicity of IMC with the complete loss of its differentiation into the layers (13% of cases were in the CCA).

http://dx.doi.org/10.5772/53445

Rate	Group 1 n=60	Group 2 n=68
Thickness of IMC of the CFA (mm)	1.32 ± 0.07	1.18 ± 0.09
The presence of atherosclerotic plaques in the arteries of the lower limbs (n/%)	57 / 95	39 / 57.4*
Thickness of IMC of CCA (mm)	1.24 ± 0,06	1.12 ± 0.08
The presence of atherosclerotic plaques in CCA (n/%)	40 / 66.7	29 / 42.6
initial indices of blood flow in the MCA		
Vps (cm/s)	75.3 ± 11.4**	79.2 ± 9.2
TAMX (cm/s)	37. 7 ± 8.5**	39.6 ± 7.63
RI	0.52 ± 0.06**	0.6 ± 0.05
indices of blood flow in the MCA after the test with breath-holding		
Vps (cm/s)	76.2 ± 12.2**	96.2 ± 10.61*
TAMX (cm/s)	38.2 ± 4.9**	57.02 ± 11.2*
RI	0.51 ±0.10**	0.55 ± 0.09*

Note: CFA - common femoral artery; CCA - common carotid artery; MCA - middle cerebral artery; Vps - Peak systolic blood flow velocity; TAMX - the time-averaged maximum velocity of blood flow; RI - index of peripheral resistance; *- $p< 0.05$ - reliability of differences between parameters obtained initially and after the test; ** - $p< 0.05$ - difference is reliable between indicators of group 1 and group 2

Table 4. Analysis of the intima-media complex of the arteries in the two groups with the assessment of cerebrovascular reactivity

Atherosclerotic vascular changes suffered by patients without DM differed from those of patients with DM. In group 2 we recorded diffuse irregular thickening of the intima-media complex with an increase of its echogenicity, sometimes with loss of differentiation of the layers mainly in large arteries (55.9% cases were in the CCA, 70.6% were in the CFA and SFA, 54.4% were in the PA, 45.6% were in the PTA and ATA), combined with abnormal thickening and the presence of atherosclerotic plaques (42.6% cases were in the CCA, 57.4% were in the CFA and SFA).

The analysis of cerebral reactivity in group 1 showed that the response on the metabolic stimulation was negative among 52 (86.7%) patients; 6 (10%) patients had a paradoxical reaction with reduced velocity parameters of the MCA.

Initial indices in group 2 did not differ significantly from the corresponding figures in group 1. However, having done breath holding test, we had a reliable increase by 16% in Vps and by 30% in TAMX ($p<0.05$). The reaction on the metabolic vasodilating test in the MCA was negative only in 5 (7.35%) cases.

These data suggest that patients with coronary heart disease and violation of carbohydrate metabolism in the peripheral blood vessels suffered the changes which had two-side and diffuse nature with many sections of lesions, whereas patients without diabetes usually had changes occurring on one side of the peripheral arteries and/or lesion of a single segment of arterial tree. We calculated a negative correlation of thickness of IMC and endothelium dependent vasodilatation ($R = -0.8743$, $p < 0.01$).

Neurohumoral disorders should be taken into account in the process of remodeling of the heart and blood vessels. Renin-angiotensin-aldosterone system (RAAS) is very important in the pathophysiological processes that eventually lead to cardiovascular remodeling, increasing the risk of cardiovascular complications [28]. Drug effect on the RAAS should be considered the standard therapeutic procedure. In this connection, study and discussion of metabolic, vascular and organ-protective effects of drugs, suppressing the activity of the RAAS are of special importance. To exclude the development of left ventricular remodeling, impaired left ventricular diastolic function and vasomotor endothelial dysfunction of the arteries from the life of patients with Type II DM is not possible. However, when treating the patients, specific efforts should be directed to slow the progression of these disorders.

We evaluated the effect of antagonist of telmisartan angiotensin II receptor on blood pressure (BP), carbohydrate and lipid metabolism, the parameters of intracardiac hemodynamics and left ventricular remodeling, endothelial vasomotor function of arteries. For 40 weeks Telmisartan - Mikardis (Boehringer Ingelheim Pharma) was prescribed to 60 patients with coronary heart disease and Type II DM in addition to standard therapy (antiplatelet, statins, peripheral vasodilators, and calcium antagonist in the pro re nata mode, oral hypoglycemic agents). The average dose for the group was 80 mg per day during the first weeks, 40 mg/day were prescribed to 24 patients during the next weeks and 36 patients took 80 mg/day).

The choice of telmisartan which is from the group of angiotensin receptor antagonists (ARA) is dictated by the results of investigations, according to which there may be a substantial difference in the influence of drugs on metabolic processes within the ARA drug group [29; 30]. This difference is explained by different ability of individual ARA to activate proliferator activation receptors by peroxisome of γ type (PPAR-γ), i.e. nuclear factors discovered by their ability to respond to xenobiotics by peroxisomal proliferation in the liver. According to Bakris G. [29], attention to PPAR is paid due to their key role in the regulation of lipid and carbohydrate metabolism in general and in the formation of insulin resistance and Type II DM in particular. The synthesis of PPAR-γ activators gives additional possibilities in the treatment of Type II DM and metabolic syndrome. However, the breadth of the spectrum of their effects allows us to think about the potential of their use in primary and secondary prevention of cardiovascular complications.

To assess the degree of compensation of carbohydrate metabolism, we measured the following indicators: levels of fasting and postprandial (2 hours after eating) blood glucose (mmol/l) at each visit, glycated hemoglobin (HbA_{1c}, %), initially and after 40 weeks of observation.

85% of patients with Type II DM and stable angina who took telmisartan in addition to standard therapy showed subjective improvement in physical condition. Having done the analysis of anginal attacks in the group, we noted a significant reduction (from 21.7 ± 2.1 to

14.3 ± 1.1 episodes) in angina attacks per week and a reduced need (from 12.8 ± 1.3 to 5.3 ± 1.1 tablets) for short-nitroglycerin per week by the 40th week of observation.

According to clinical measurements of blood pressure (BP) a significant reduction in office systolic (SBP) blood pressure and diastolic blood pressure (DBP) was observed among patients being treated with telmisartan during the test appearances, 95% of patients having target BP level of SBP. Target BP level of DBP was in 96.7% cases, $p < 0.05$.

According to the ambulatory blood pressure monitoring (ABPM), abnormal profile of blood pressure trend was observed among 88.3% of patients, most of them (75%) forming the category of "non-dippers" (patients with lack of normal physiological reduction in blood pressure at night). However, we identified cases of distorted circadian rhythm with a predominantly nocturnal hypertension (13.3%), i.e. the group of "night-pickers".

After 40 weeks of the therapy we received reduction in daily average SBP and DBP, time index of hypertension for 24 hours, the variability in SBP and DBP ($p<0.05$) (Table 5).

We observed a normalization of circadian BP profile among 85% of patients that was 96.2% of patients with abnormal circadian rhythm (non-dipper and night-picker). Therapy with telmisartan allowed us to reduce indicators of the magnitude and rate of morning increase in BP. Thus, the magnitude of morning increase in SBP decreased by 49% and the magnitude of morning increase in DBP decreased by 51.4% while the rate of morning increase in SBP decreased by 69% and the rate of morning increase in DBP decreased by 62.9% ($p<0,03$).

Rate	Initial	After 40 weeks
circadian blood pressure monitoring indicators		
Daily average SBP (mmHg)	148.4 ± 11.3*	127.1 ± 3.3
Daily average DBP (mmHg)	89.3 ± 6.7*	77.2 ± 3.1
The daily variability of SBP (mmHg)	21.9 ± 2.8*	15.2 ± 1.7
The daily variability of DBP (mmHg)	16.4 ± 2.3*	9.9 ± 1.1
Time index of systolic hypertension in 24 hours (%)	80.4 ± 5.3*	32.3 ± 5.2
Time index of diastolic hypertension in 24 hours (%)	66.7 ± 3.4*	22.3 ± 2.5
The rate morning increase of SBP (mmHg/h)	29.7 ± 3.2	9.2 ± 1.4
The rate morning increase of DBP (mmHg/h)	17.8 ± 3.1	6.6 ± 1.0
circadian ECG monitoring indicators		
DMI (min)	45.3 ± 3.2*	20.7± 1.4
PEMI (min)	14.7 ± 2.5	11.3 ± 1.3
SMI (min)	31.1 ± 2.1*	9.5 ± 1.5

Note: differences were significant between the numerical values of initial rates and rates after 40 weeks of therapy with telmisartan.

Table 5. Dynamics of functional parameters during therapy with telmisartan

We indicated the positive dynamics of indicators characterizing the process of left ventricular remodeling: a decrease in end-diastolic volume (EDV) and end-systolic volume (ESV) by 7.5% and 8.4%, respectively, and an increase in ejection fraction by 6.6%, $p<0.05$. The fraction of systolic shortening of the anterior-posterior size of the left ventricular increased by 8.2%.

Daily rates of myocardial ischemia have undergone significant changes: number of ischemic episodes decreased from 4.8±0.34 to 2.3±0.3; maximum depth of ST segment depression decreased from 2.5 ± 0.2 mm to 1.7 ± 0.1 mm; duration of ischemic episodes decreased from 45.3±3.2 min to 20.7 ± 1.4 min. We should emphasize that the positive dynamics was indicated in most cases when we analyzed data on silent myocardial ischemia: duration of all episodes of silent myocardial ischemia decreased during the day ($p<0.05$) and the number of episodes of silent myocardial ischemia decreased from 2.8±0.4 to 1.2±0.2 per day too.

We explain the result obtained not only by improved circadian BP profile and adequate control, but also by the presumable ability of the drug to effect myocardial blood flow making coronary vasodilation and redistributing blood flow towards the subendocardial layers of myocardium, which are particularly vulnerable to ischemia. We established the correlation of the duration of painless ST segment depression and a daily index of SBP ($R= -0.53$, $p<0.02$), daily index of DBP ($R= -0.61$, $p<0.03$).

These reactive hyperemia tests allowed us to indicate the improvement of vasomotor function induced by shear stress, endothelium dependent vasodilatation increasing from 3.7±1.1% to 7.2±1.1%. We had positive dynamics of velocity indicators: peak systolic blood flow velocity increased from 0.84±0.06 m/s to 0.94±0.04 m/s ($p<0.05$); maximum diastolic blood flow velocity increased from 0.13±0.03 m/s to 0.18±0.03 m/s ($p<0.05$); time-averaged maximum flow velocity increased from 0.29±0.06 to 0.46±0.04 ($p<0.05$).

Individual analysis of the endothelium dependent vasodilatation dynamics during treatment with telmisartan showed that the number of patients with impaired endothelial function decreased to 51.7%, while the number of persons with pathological vasoconstriction/vasodilation in the absence of performing the test with reactive hyperemia decreased by 23.3% (Figure 3.).

Recovery of adequate dilatation response of vessels to reactive hyperemia test is a necessary link in the chain of effective therapeutic intervention aimed at reducing of cardiovascular risk. It is known that activation of the RAAS is an indispensable part of the pathogenesis of endothelial dysfunction, so the use of these drugs in its correction seems most reasonable at present. The mechanism of endothelial function improvement by drugs blocking the RAAS is explained at present by the elimination of the adverse effects of ATII [31; 32] having a powerful vasoconstriction influence by stimulating of AT1-receptor of vascular smooth muscle cells. It is also considered as an inducer of oxidative stress with production of superoxide anion by simulation of nicotinamide-adenine-dinucleotide-phosphate; the action of angiotensin II is opposite to the action of nitric oxide, i.e. oxidase.

http://dx.doi.org/10.5772/53445

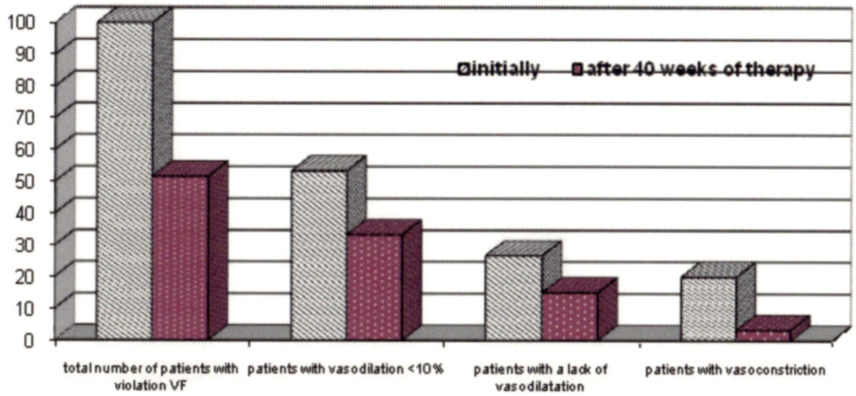

Note: The data are presented in percents, VF - vasomotor function.

Figure 3. Correction of endothelial vasomotor dysfunction of arteries during the course therapy with telmisartan.

We also associate the resulting effect of telmisartan to improve vasomotor endothelial function with the complicated mechanism of regulation of the circadian blood pressure variability. In this sense, control of blood pressure with ARA group drugs can be considered reasonable in terms of impact on the pathophysiological mechanisms leading to the morning increase of BP, and in terms of protection of patients at the beginning of drug action during the regular morning drug intake. This fact may be proved by revealed correlation dependence of the endothelium dependent vasodilatation dynamics from the time index of hypertension on DBP for 24 hours ($R= -0.64$, $p<0.003$) and the daily index ($R= 0.54$, $p<0.02$).

Conducting therapy with telmisartan, we noted a significant decrease in glycated hemoglobin level from 8.41±0.2% to 6.5±0.4%, a decrease of fasting plasma glucose from 8.72±0.35 mmol/l to 6.67±0.4 mmol/l ($p<0.02$) and a decrease of postprandial blood glucose level from 9.2±1.68 to 8.5±1.38 mmol/l ($p<0.05$). The number of patients who achieved compensation of carbohydrate metabolism in three indices of "glycemic triad" rose from 10% to 23.3%. We indicated the correlation dependence of endothelium dependent vasodilation dynamics from glycated hemoglobin ($R= -0.56$, $p <0.05$).

We evaluated the dynamics of lipid metabolism indices among patients with Type II DM during therapy with telmisartan. After 40 weeks we noted an improvement of laboratory parameters which showed a decrease in total cholesterol by 23%, low-density lipoprotein cholesterol by 21%, triglycerides by 26% ($p<0.05$). We explain it by the increase in sensitivity of tissues to insulin and decreased hyperinsulinemia, which largely determine the metabolism of lipids in the body.

The data obtained allow us to state that telmisartan has a positive metabolic effect, which has an additional metabolic effect along with mechanisms of local pancreatic RAAS blocking being common for all the ARA drugs [33], i.e. agonistic effect on PPAR-◎-receptors, which control the activity of cytokines - the regulators of intercellular interactions, leading to a positive influence on carbohydrate and lipid metabolism and reduction of severity of insulin resistance (IR) phenomenon.

4. The conclusion

So, patients with coronary heart disease and Type II DM had silent myocardial ischemia 2 times more often than patients with coronary heart disease who had no disorders of carbohydrate metabolism. Patients with coronary heart disease and Type II DM had dominating daily duration of episodes of myocardial ischemia and a maximum depth of ST segment depression. Besides, they had reduced endothelium-dependent vasodilation reaction (endothelium-dependent vasodilation =3.7±1.1%). Violation of the functional state of the vascular endothelium correlates with the registration frequency ($R= -0.68$, $p<0.05$) and duration of episodes of silent myocardial ischemia ($R= -0.53$, $p<0.01$). Endothelial dysfunction of the coronary arteries which is manifested by blood vessels inability to adequate increase in conditions of increased myocardial oxygen demand has an influence on the genesis and progression of ischemia.

The results obtained during our research prove that metabolic factors play a significant role in the development of endothelial dysfunction. To predict vascular complications it is necessary to assess vasomotor function of arteries endothelium among patients with Type II DM.

Prescribing receptor antagonists of angiotensin II, we take into account organ-protective effects of drugs, manifested by the selective blockade of the tissue RAAS and indirect stimulation of the AT_2-receptors during their long-term intake.

It is considered to be a proved fact [34; 35] that the increased activity of tissue RAAS causes long-term effects of angiotensin II (AII), which are manifested in structural and functional changes in target organs and lead to the development of a number of pathological processes such as hypertrophy, miofibroz, atherosclerotic lesion of vessels. The research [36] showed that a human body had alternative ways with chymase, cathepsin G, serine proteases in addition to ACE-dependent pathway of conversion of angiotensin I to angiotensin II. According to Elmfeldt D. and colleagues [37], chymase dependent formation of AII prevails in myocardial interstitium and adventitia and media of vessels, whereas ACE-dependent formation prevails in blood plasma. This fact explains the risk of AII escape phenomenon during the long-term intake of ACE (angiotensin-converting enzyme).

Additional metabolic effect of selective antagonist of AT1-receptor of telmisartan is agonistic effect on PPAR-◎-receptors, which is manifested in a significantly improved glucose and lipid profiles indices. This effect allows us to consider it as the drug of choice in the treatment of patients suffering a combination of metabolic disorders, hypertension in clinical manifestations of stable angina. Correlation analysis showed the dependence of HbA1c on the daily duration of ST depression episodes ($R=0.66$, $p<0.01$) and the duration of asymptomatic ST depression ($R=0.75$, $p<0.02$).

Modern methods in treatment of patients with coronary heart disease and DM allow using a scheme of the multi-component therapy, in which much attention is given to the improvement of endothelial function. It leads to the concurrent positive therapeutic effects of telmisartan on major links in the chain of cardiovascular complications in Type II DM improving glucose and blood lipid profile indices, a more pronounced organ protective effect. In addition, it directly prevents the development of ischemia and its main clinical manifestation.

Summary

The development of ischemic episodes in the absence of pain or angina equivalents (e.g., dyspnea, arrhythmias) is possible when a patient has coronary heart disease. Atypical clinical course makes diagnosis of coronary insufficiency with disorders of carbohydrate metabolism rather difficult. Having done the analysis of the daily trend of ST segment and the diary records of patients with DM we have identified a silent myocardial ischemia in 93.3% cases, 60% patients having a combination of painful and painless episodes of myocardial ischemia. 33.3% from 93.3% cases of ischemic episodes of ST segment depression were not accompanied by any subjective symptoms. Patients with coronary heart disease and DM have reduced endothelium-dependent vasodilation reaction (endothelium-dependent vasodilation =3.7±1.1%). Violation of the functional state of the vascular endothelium correlates with the registration frequency ($R= -0.68$, $p<0.05$) and duration of episodes of silent myocardial ischemia ($R= -0.53$, $p<0.01$).

Abbreviations

ABPM - ambulatory blood pressure monitoring

ARA - angiotensin receptor antagonists

ATII - angiotensin II

BP - blood pressure

CHD - Coronary Heart Disease

CHF - chronic heart failure

DM - Diabetes Mellitus

DB2 - Type 2 Diabetes Mellitus

ECG – electrocardiogram

ED - endothelial dysfunction

FC - Functional Class

IMC - Intima-Media Complex

IR - insulin resistance

NO - Nitrogen Oxide
PEMI - Painful Episode of Myocardial Ischemia
PPAR - peroxisome proliferator activating ◉-receptor
RAAS - Renin-angiotensin-aldosterone system

Author details

I.P. Tatarchenko, N.V. Pozdnyakova, O.I. Morozova, A.G. Mordovina, S.A. Sekerko and I.A. Petrushin

Penza Extension Course Institute for Medical Practitioners, Russia

References

[1] Zarich, S. W, & Nesto, R. W. Diabetic cardiomyopathy. Am Heart J (1989). , 118(5), 1000-12.

[2] Killip, T. Silent Myocardial Ischemia: Some good news. Circulation (1997). , 95, 1992-93.

[3] Cohn, P. F, & Fox, K. M. Silent myocardial ischemia. Circulation (2003). , 108, 1263-90.

[4] Schoenenberger, A. W, Jamshidi, P, Kobza, R, et al. Progression of coronary artery disease during long-term follow-up of the Swiss Interventional Study on Silent Ischemia Type II (SWISSI II). Clin. Cardiol (2010). , 33(5), 289-95.

[5] Jermendy, G, & Davidovits, Z. Khoor S: Silent coronary artery disease in diabetic patients with cardiac autonomic neuropathy. Diabetes Care (1994). , 17, 1231-32.

[6] Gokcel, A, Aydin, M, & Yalcin, F. Silent coronary artery disease in patients with type 2 diabetes mellitus. Acta Diabetol (2003). , 40, 176-80.

[7] Kempler, P. Neuropathies. Pathomechanism, clinical presentation, diagnosis, therapy/ Ed. by P. Kempler. Springer; (2002).

[8] Dzau, V, Bernstein, K, Celermajer, D, et al. Pathophysiologic and therapeutic implications of tissue ACE: a consensus report. Cardiovasc Drugs Ther (2002). , 16(2), 149-60.

[9] Celermajer, D. S. Endothelial dysfunction: does it matter? Is it relevant? J Amer Coll Cardiology (1997). , 30, 325-33.

[10] Antonetti, D. A, Barber, A. J, Lieth, E, et al. Vascular permeability in experimental diabetes is associated with reduced endothelial occludin content: occludin expression is decreased in experimental diabetic retinopathy. Diabetes (1998). , 47, 1953-59.

[11] Bassenge, E, & Zanziger, J. Nitrates in different vascular beds, nitrate tolerance, and interactions with endothelial function. Am. J. Cardiol (1992). , 28, 371-74.

[12] Cacoub, P, Dorent, R, Nataf, P, et al. Endothelin-1 in the lungs of patients with pulmonary hypertension. Cardiovasc Res (1997). , 33(1), 196-200.

[13] Kario, K, Matsuo, T, Kobayashi, H, et al. Hyperinsulinemia and hemostatic abnormalities are associated with silent lacunar cerebral infarcts in elderly hypertensive subjects. J Am Coll Cardiol (2001). , 37, 871-77.

[14] Luscher, T, Wenzel, R. R, & Noll, G. Local regulation of the coronary circulation in health and disease: role of nitric oxide and endothelin. Europ Heart J (1995). Suppl. C): , 51-58.

[15] Cipolla, M. Diabetes and Endothelial Dysfunction: A Clinical Perspective. Endocr Rev (2001). , 22(1), 36-52.

[16] Vanhoutte, P. M, & Boulanger, C. M. Endotheliumdependent responses in hypertension. Hypertens Res (1995). , 18(2), 87-98.

[17] Tooke, J. E. The association between insulin resistance and endotheliopathy. Diab Obes Metab (1999). , 1, 23-31.

[18] Folli, F, Saad, M. J, Velloso, L, et al. Crosstalk between insulin and angiotensin II signaling systems. Exp Clin Endocrinol Diabetes (1999). , 107, 133-39.

[19] Ceriello, A, Cavarape, A, Martinelli, L, et al. The post-prandial state in type 2 diabetes and endothelial dysfunction: effects of insulin aspart. Diabet Med (2004). , 21, 171-75.

[20] Hinderliter, A. L, & Caugher, M. Assessing endothelial function as a risk factor for cardiovascular disease. Curr Atheroscler Rep (2003). , 5(6), 506-13.

[21] Schachinger, V, Britten, M. B, & Zeiher, A. M. Prognostic impact of coronary vasodilator dysfunction on adverse long-term outcome of coronary heart disease. Circulation (2000). , 101, 1899-906.

[22] Celermajer, D. S, & Sorensen, K. E. Non-invasive detection of endothelial dysfunction in children and adults at risk of atherosclerosis. Lancet (1992). , 340, 1111-15.

[23] Lelyuk, V. G, & Lelyuk, S. E. The technique of ultrasound examination of the vascular system: scanning technology and regulatory indicators. Textbook: (2002).

[24] Campbell, I. Type 2 diabetes mellitus: «The silent killer». Practical Diabetes Int (2001). , 18(6), 187-91.

[25] Suwaidi, J. A, Hamasaki, S, Higano, S. T, et al. Long-term follow-up of patients with mild coronary artery disease and endothelial dysfunction. Circulation (2000). , 101, 948-54.

[26] Zateyshchikova, A. A, & Zateyshchikov, D. A. Endothelial regulation of vascular tone: setting, and clinical significance. Cardiology (1998). , 9, 68-80.

[27] Tatarchenko, I. P, Pozdnyakova, N. V, Mordovina, A. G, & Morozova, O. I. Dysfunction of vascular endothelium in the evaluation of episodes of myocardial ischemia in type 2 diabetes. Problems of Endocrinology (2009). , 6, 7-11.

[28] Dzau, V. The cardiovascular continuum and rennin-angiotensin-aldosterone system blocade. Hypertens J (2005). Suppl): , 9-17.

[29] Bakris, G. Comparison of telmisartan vs. valsartan in the treatment of mild to moderate hypertension using ambulatory blood pressure monitoring. J Clin Hypertension (2002). Suppl. 1): 26-31.

[30] Velliquette, R. A, & Ernsberger, P. Contrasting metabolic effects of antihypertensive agents. J Pharmacol Exp Ther (2003). , 307, 1104-11.

[31] Dedov, E. E, & Aleksandrov, A. A. Diabetes mellitus and AT1-receptor antagonists: in search of solution. Russian Journal of Medicine (2005). , 11, 11-16.

[32] Karalliedde, J, & Viberti, G. Evidence for renoprotection by blockade of the renin-angiotensin-aldosterone system in hypertension and diabetes. J Hum Med (2006). , 35, 890-99.

[33] Lau, T, Carlsson, P. O, & Leung, P. S. Evidence for local angiotensin-generating system and dose-dependent inhibition of glucose-stimulated insulin release by angiotensin II in isolated pancreatic islets. Diabetologia (2004). , 47, 240-48.

[34] Chung, O, & Unger, T. Angiotensin II receptor blockade and end organ protection. Amer J Hypertension (1999). , 12, 150-56.

[35] Tatarchenko, I. P, Pozdnyakova, N. V, Mordovina, A. G, Morozova, O. I, Sekerko, S. A, & Petrushin, I. A. Clinical and functional assessment of organ-protective effectiveness of enalapril and telmisartan among patients with hypertension. Cardiology (2011). , 4, 16-21.

[36] Burnier, M, & Brunner, H. Angiotensin II receptor antagonists. Lancet (2000). , 355, 637-45.

[37] Elmfeld, D, Olofsson, B, & Meredith, P. The relationships between dose and antihypertensive effect of four AT1-receptor blockers. Differenc in potency and efficacy. Blood Pressure (2002). , 11, 293-301.

Chapter 4

Sex Differences in Sudden Cardiac Death

Anastasia Susie Mihailidou, Rebecca Ritchie and
Anthony W. Ashton

Additional information is available at the end of the chapter

http://dx.doi.org/10.5772/55631

1. Introduction

Ischemic heart disease continues to be the leading cause of death in most countries and a major health burden, with approximately 50% of deaths due to sudden cardiac death (SCD) [Zipes & Wellens, 1998; Wong et al. 2001; Mazeika 2001]. The increasing prevalence of diabetes will also impact on SCD incidence. Patients with either type 1 or type 2 diabetes have significantly higher mortality and morbidity following acute myocardial infarction (AMI) than do the rest of the population. Other conditions such as hypertension, hypertrophic cardiomyopathy, aortic stenosis and aging may also increase the risk of SCD. Sex differences in prevalence and clinical outcomes are recognised [Bairey et al. 2006; Wake et al. 2007], although many randomized clinical trials do not have adequate numbers of women to allow sex-specific analyses [Xhyheri & Bugiardini 2010; Melloni et al. 2010]. Ischemic heart disease is the primary cause of death for women at all ages, with annual mortality rates for women 35-55 years greater than breast cancer [Bell et al. 2000] and approximately 81% of deaths in low- and middle-income countries [Mosca et al. 2011]. The incidence of SCD differs according to geographical region depending on the prevalence of coronary or ischemic heart disease [Priori et al. 2001]. In the United States, during 1989 to 1998, there was markedly less of a decline in SCD rates among women than for men - women aged 35 to 44 years had a 21% increased SCD rate compared with a 2.8% decline for men of the same age group [Zheng et al. 2001]. During the same period, women were dying of a cardiac arrest before hospital arrival (52%) compared with 42% for men [Shaw et al. 2006]. Compared to males women are generally older when presenting with AMI [Canto et al. 2012] and with women's longer life expectancy, the estimates are expected to rise even further in future decades. Although risk factors for IHD and SCD are often assumed to be similar in women and men, there are also differences. For instance, SCD will occur before any other signs of coronary heart disease in women [de Vreede-Swagemakers et al. 1997; Kannel et al. 1998; Albert et al. 2003] whereas ventricular dysrhythmias following AMI, contribute to increased risk in men but not women [Dahlberg, 1990; Kim et al. 2001]. There may are also be differences in mechanisms for SCD between older and premenopausal or middle aged women. This chapter will review the sex differences in mechanism of SCD and possible treatment strategies.

2. Ischemic heart disease and sudden cardiac death

Cardiovascular disease (CVD) is the primary cause of death globally with 17.3 million deaths in 2008, representing approximately 50% of non-communicable disease deaths [World Health Report (WHO), 2012]. Of these deaths, approximately 7.3 million (42%) were due to ischemic heart disease (IHD). Figure 1 shows the proportion of IHD deaths according to income status (data adapted from WHO Report 2012]. In middle- and high-income countries, IHD was the primary cause of deaths, whereas it was fourth highest in low-income countries. In the United States, coronary heart disease (CHD) resulted in 1 of every 6 deaths in 2008. According to the recent American Heart Association report [Roger et al. 2012], there is a coronary event approximately every 25 seconds, and approximately one death every minute. More women (64%) than men (50%) die suddenly of coronary heart disease without any previous symptoms of this disease, while people with previous AMI have sudden death rates 4 to 6 times that of the general population [Roger et al. 2012].

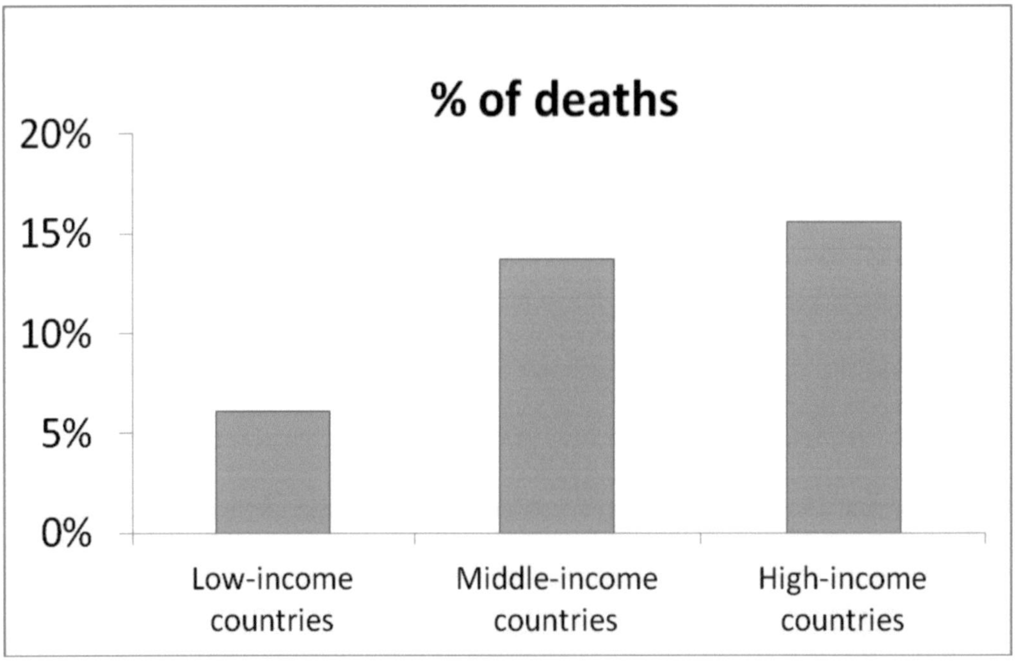

Figure 1. Ischemic heart disease deaths according to income status

The prevalence of SCD varies depending on the definition used between different studies. Another confounder is that many sudden deaths are not witnessed, and without cardiac monitoring at the time of death. Prevalence may vary from 13% when SCD is defined as death suddenly or unexpectedly within an hour of onset of symptoms, to 18.5% of all deaths when this period is extended to 24 hours after onset of symptoms [de Vreede-Swagemakers et al. 1997]. Most studies report that SCD results from a fatal cardiac arrhythmia, either degeneration of ventricular tachycardia (VT) into ventricular fibrillation(VF), leading to disorganized ventricular contraction or severe bradycardia or pulseless electrical activity [Lane et al. 2005]. Ventricular arrhythmias have been documented in 85% of patients with severe congestive heart failure [Singh et al. 1997]. Dilated nonischemic and hypertrophic cardiomyopathies contribute to the next largest number of SCDs, whereas other cardiac disorders, including congenital heart defects and genetically determined ion channel anomalies, contribute 5–10% of SCDs [Lane et al. 2005].

3. Risk factors for sudden cardiac death

To determine the risk factors for SCD many studies examine the same traditional factors associated with IHD, which include systolic blood pressure, dyslipidemia, smoking, obesity, heavy alcohol consumption, diabetes mellitus and age [Kannel et al. 1985; Jouven et al. 1999; Khot et al. 2003; Sandhu et al. 2012], summarised in Table 1. Subjects with inherited arrhythmogenic disorders such as long-QT syndrome and Brugada syndrome are also at increased risk for SCD. Similar risk factors for men and women were identified in the Framingham Study which compared 2873 women with 2336 men aged 30 to 62 years [Schatzkln et al.1984; Kannel et al. 1998]. Similar to IHD, the presence of hypertension and diabetes increased the risk of SCD at all ages, whereas at all ages, sudden death risk ratios associated with diabetes were greater in women than men. Interestingly, the risk factors of hematocrit and vital capacity, predicted SCD in women but not men [Schatzkln et al. 1984]. Risk factors may also differ between premenopausal and older women. For instance, coronary heart disease (CHD) death in premenopausal women is due to plaque erosions with minimal coronary artery narrowing, whereas older women have high cholesterol levels and plaque rupture, with severe coronary artery narrowing [Canto et al. 2012].

As noted in Table 1, the risk factors for SCD are not consistently recorded and ventricular ectopy is one risk factor which is omitted since some of the deaths may have occurred in the absence of monitoring. Trials which have targeted only suppressing this ectopy to prevent SCD have not been successful and possibly hazardous [Akiyama et al. 1991]. Parental history of MI before age 60 years has also been identified as a risk factor for SCD, but only among women younger than age 60 years. The traditional factors for IHD also elevate the risk of SCD by 2- to 4-fold and include hypertension, diabetes and smoking [Albert et al. 2003]. Smoking was identified as a strong risk factor for SCD among young women (<60 years). Since it is a modifiable risk factor, Sandhu and colleagues (2012) recently reported a prospective study showing that smoking cessation significantly reduced and eliminated excess SCD risk [Sandhu et al. 2012].

	Age (yr)		M:F	High cholesterol		Prior CHD (%)		Hypertension		Diabetes		Smoking	
	M	F	%	M	F	without	with	M	F	M	F	M	F
Kannel et al. (1998)*		30-62	45:55			44M:63F	56M:37F						
35-64 yr				1.3	1.4			1.9	1.7	3.9	1.5	1	1.4
65-94 yr				1	1.4			2.2	1.7	4	1.3	0.9	1.2
Schatzkln et al. (1984)	30-62	30-62	45:55										
Without prior CHD								135±21	137±25				
With prior CHD								143±24	158±29				
Albert et al. (2003)	-	30- 55	100F		1.33				3.17		4.9		
Parental history of MI		1.87 (<60)											
		1.36 ("/ >60)											
Shaw et al. (2006)								↑	-	-	↑	↑	
Age threshold	≥45	≥55											
Family History of CHD	<55	<65											
Khot et al (2003)	59.9 (11.6)	66.1 (11.2)		34%	40%			38.4%	55.9%	15.3 %	23.2 %	29.5 %	41.6 %

M= males and F= females; *Same cohort as Schatzkln et al. (1984)

Table 1. Relative risk for factors associated with Sudden Cardiac Death

In considering risk factors for IHD and SCD, one cannot overlook how endogenous levels of sex hormones may be contributing. Men and women show differences in ECG repolarization with QT prolongation in women, while male hearts from many species are hypertrophied relative to female hearts [Marsh et al. 1998]. In premenopausal women with normal ovulation, estrogen and other endogenous hormones provide cardioprotection and lower incidence of IHD compared to age-matched men. In contrast, during menopause, there is a fall in estrogen levels to approximately one-tenth that of premenopausal levels [Paoletti et al. 1997] and estrone, produced by peripheral conversion of androgens in the adipose tissue, is the main estrogen. In the Women's Ischemia Syndrome Evaluation (WISE) Study premenopausal women that had a stress-induced disruption in ovulatory cycling with resulting low levels of estrogen had a 7.4-fold increased risk of obstructive coronary artery disease [Shaw et al. 2006]. Although there is increased focus on the lack of estrogen, the role of androgens should also be considered, given that they activate atherosclerotic-related genes in men but not women and activate androgen receptors in cardiac myocytes of both men and women, to produce hypertrophy [Marsh et al. 1999].

The risk factors for IHD common in postmenopausal women, include obesity, hypertension, and dyslipidemia. Menopausal women also have a greater loss in physical functioning compared to men [Poehlman 2002], which aggravates weight gain, insulin resistance, and hypertension [Shaw et al. 2006]. Loss of ovarian estrogen during menopause is also associated with redistribution of abdominal fat, further increasing the risk of IHD [Lamon-Fava et al. 1996]. The role of hormone replacement therapy (HRT) for postmenopausal women has been controversial. This is due to conflicting results from observational trials performed prior to 2002 which showed a reduction in risk of cardiovascular disease, osteoporosis, and colon cancer whereas large randomized clinical trials such as the Women's Health Initiative showed no cardiovascular benefit from hormone replacement therapy [Schierbeck et al. 2012]. The timing of initiating hormone therapy has been suggested as a possible explanation for these conflicting results. The observational studies started hormone therapy shortly after menopause, whereas the large randomised studies, which showed no or negative cardiovascular effects, initiated hormone therapy 5 to 20 years after menopause. The recent prospective, multicentre, HRT study, the Danish Osteoporosis Prevention Study (DOPS) was initiated to evaluate HRT as primary prevention for osteoporotic fractures [Schierbeck et al. 2012]. Healthy, recently postmenopausal women (within 7 months) aged 45-58 were recruited to the study and were randomly allocated to receive HRT or no treatment (control). Treatment ceased after 11 years although participants were followed for death, cardiovascular disease, and cancer for a further 5 years (total 16 years).Following 10 years randomised treatment, women receiving HRT early after menopause had significantly reduced risk of mortality, heart failure, or myocardial infarction, without any increase in risk of cancer, venous thromboembolism, or stroke.

4. Mechanism of sudden cardiac death

Sustained VT and VF are responsible for at least two thirds of sudden cardiac deaths [Huikuri et al. 2001] with sex-differences in arrhythmic SCD reported [Orencia et al. (1993); Kannel et al. (1998); Zheng et al. (2001); Abildstrom et al. (2002); Adabag et al. (2008); Verheugt et al. (2008)]. Pre-existing coronary heart disease significantly contributes to SCD in men [Lane et al. 2005] whereas women are 66% less likely to be diagnosed with coronary heart disease before SCD [Albert et al. 1996; Chiuve et al. (2011)]. Several studies have investigated whether sex disparities in the risk factors for SCD may contribute to these differences. Atherogenic risk factors were found to be predictive in men but not women. Similarly, asymptomatic ventricular dysrhythmias are an independent risk for death in men but have not been shown to be a risk for women [Dahlberg, 1990]. Patients with congestive heart failure due to cardiomyopathy or ischemic heart disease have the highest rate of SCD, although the contributing factors remain poorly defined. Recent studies have suggested that genetic or environmental factors may predispose to fatal ventricular arrhythmia, particularly in women. However, mutations or rare variants in the cardiac sodium channel SCN5A were found in <2% cases screened and further studies are required [Albert et al. 2008]. Stress cardiomyopathy, also known as takotsubo cardiomyopathy, transient apical ballooning or broken heart syndrome is found predominantly in postmenopausal women [Nef et al. 2010]. Emotional or physical stress trigger symptom onset, which is similar to those in AMI, including sudden onset of chest pain associated with ST-segment elevation, and moderate increases in creatine kinase and troponin levels. Prognosis for stress cardiomyopathy is favorable, although fatal complications may occur, including cardiogenic shock, malignant arrhythmias and left ventricular free wall rupture.

Cardiac remodelling following either ischemia or AMI initially develops to compensate for failing cardiac function with evidence of hypertrophy, cardiomyocyte apoptosis, inflammation and fibrosis. Initially these changes are beneficial but ultimately transition to deteriorating cardiac function and lead to heart failure [Abel et al. 2008]. Although left ventricular (LV) dysfunction significantly increases the risk of SCD [Anand et al. 2006; Stecker et al. 2006], other risk factors need to be considered since women are 50% less likely to exhibit severe LV dysfunction, with structurally normal hearts identified at autopsy [Chugh et al. 2003]. Alternative mechanisms of SCD therefore need to be considered, given that women with coronary heart disease have significantly lower risk for SCD.

The renin-angiotensin-aldosterone system (RAAS) plays a significant role in ischemic heart disease and AMI and blockade of this system has emerged as an important therapeutic intervention. Elevated plasma aldosterone levels are an independent risk factor for mortality during AMI [Beygui et al. 2006; Palmer et al. 2008] and are predictive of cardiovascular events in acute coronary syndrome in the presence or absence of AMI [Tomaschitz et al. 2010]. Aldosterone exerts its actions by interacting with its receptor, the mineralocorticoid receptor (MR) or "aldosterone" receptor. Both aldosterone and the physiological glucocorticoids (cortisol (humans)/corticosterone (rodents), which are at 100-fold higher circulating levels bind to the MR. Selective activation of MR in target tissues is achieved by co-expression of the enzyme 11β-hydroxysteroid dehydrogenase type 2 (11β-HDS2). In contrast with vascular and renal tissues, 11βHSD2 is not expressed in cardiomyocytes [Sheppard & Autelitano 2002], and therefore endogenous glucocorticoids normally do not mimic aldosterone, but act as MR antagonists [Gomez et al 1990; Sato & Funder, 1996; Young & Funder, 1996]. Redox regulation has been shown to modulate glucocorticoid hormone action *in vivo* [Makino et al. 1999] and expression of oestrogen receptors [Tamir et al. 2002]. For every molecule of cortisol converted to cortisone, one molecule of the pyridine nucleotide NAD is reduced to NADH. Since NADH has been shown to activate corepressors for other transcription factors in various systems [Zhang et al. 2002; Fjeld et al. 2003], and changes in redox state may determine cardiomyocyte MR activation by glucocorticoids [Mihailidou et al. 2009].

Elevated aldosterone levels promote electrical remodelling through activation of MR or "aldosterone" receptors, thus potentially increasing the incidence of sudden cardiac death. In experimental studies, aldosterone has a direct effect on cardiomyocyte calcium [Ouvrard-

Pascaud et al. 2005] and sodium [Mihailidou et al. 2000] as well as producing hypokalemia and hypomagnesemia [Mihailidou et al. 2002]. These electrolyte imbalances have been translated clinically with the Framingham Heart Study showing that low serum concentrations of potassium and magnesium were linked to increased risk of SCD. A decrease in potassium of 0.48 mEq/litre or magnesium of 0.16 mEq/litre level was associated with a 27% (C.I. 6% - 51%) and a 20% (C.I. 3% - 41%) greater odds of complex or frequent ventricular premature contractions [Tsuji et al. 1994].

Possible other targets include the gap junction connexins and identifying whether they are regulated differently between males and females. Connexins allow rapid and coordinated electrical excitation and facilitate intercellular exchange of small molecules. Experimental studies have shown that normal gap junction expression and phosphorylation in the heart is essential for organized myocellular electrical activity [Stauffer et al. 2011]. Interestingly female hearts have higher levels of cardiac connexin 43 (Cx43) [Tribulova et al. 2005] and lower lethal arrhythmia susceptibility [Knezl et al. 2008]. Further studies are required to confirm whether abnormalities in cardiac Cx43 expression and phosphorylation are the primary trigger of arrhythmogenesis, since this occurs prior to other structural remodelling changes [Stauffer et al. 2011].

Recent studies have explored the role of microRNAs (miRNAs) in many biological and pathological processes and the role of circulating miRNAs as sensitive biomarkers with aberrant expression of miRNA directly reflecting disease state. Ai and colleagues (2010), recently found upregulated cardiac miR-1 in an animal model of AMI, with similar increases in plasma in patients with AMI. These increased miR-1 levels correlated with abnormal QRS widening in AMI [Ai et al. 2010]. Over-expression of miR-1 has been shown to induce and aggravate arrhythmogenesis. The mechanism proposed is by impairing cardiac conduction by post-transcriptional repression of KCNJ2 that encodes the inward rectifier K+ channel subunit Kir2.1 and GJA1 which encode connexin 43 gap junction channels [Yang et al. 2007].

5. Treatment strategies

Primary prevention of SCD continues to be a public health challenge since most deaths are among people who were not identified as high risk prior to the event. Implantable cardiovert-er–defibrillator (ICD) therapy is the current recommended treatment strategy for high risk patients with severe left ventricular dysfunction (Sudden Cardiac Death in Heart Failure Trial (SCDHeFT), [Bardy et al. 2005]. Subgroup analysis in SCDHeFT as well as in another primary prevention trial, the Defibrillators in Nonischemic Cardiomyopathy Treatment Evaluation (DEFINITE) [Kadish et al. 2004] suggested that women may receive less benefit from ICD therapy than men. Interestingly in both these large trials, only 24%-30% of participants and since women have a lower incidence of VF compared to men [Kim et al. 2001; Wigginton et al. 2002] and therefore may not have been adequately powered to determine the influence of gender on outcome for ICD therapy.

ICDs treat (but do not prevent) the ventricular arrhythmias and therefore increased morbidity remains. ICD therapy is rarely considered where LV function is preserved, except in specific conditions with increased SCD risk such as hypertrophic obstructive cardiomyopathy, long QT and Brugada syndromes, and idiopathic VF [DiMarco 2003]. A community-based study conducted by Stecker and colleagues (2006) showed that only 30% of patients that died from SCD previously had sufficiently decreased LV systolic function to meet the criteria for ICD implantation. Patients with normal LV systolic function were generally younger, predominantly female and less likely to have an established diagnosis of coronary heart disease. Since ICDs treat the arhythmia but not prevent the underlying cause, there is a need to find new treatment strategies that target the cellular mechanisms involved. Standard antiarrhythmic medication has not reduced (and in some cases, has increased), the incidence of SCD [Lane et al. 2005]. Suitable adjunct treatment in the primary and secondary prevention of SCD includes beta blockers and non-anti-arrhythmic agents, i.e., those that do not directly target the electrophysiological action in cardiac muscle or specialized conduction system, such as angiotensin converting enzyme inhibitors (ACEI), angiotensin receptor–blockers, lipid-lowering agents, aldosterone or MR antagonists, thrombolytic and antithrombotic agents [Lane et al. 2005].

It is worth considering the role of aldosterone or MR blockade for both primary prevention of SCD for those at high-risk and as an adjunct therapy based on the important findings from the large randomized clinical studies, the Randomized ALdactone Evaluation Study (RALES) [Pitt et al. 1999] and the Eplerenone Post–Acute Myocardial Infarction Heart Failure Efficacy and Survival Study (EPHESUS) [Pitt et al. 2003], which showed a significant reduction in SCD. The first of these trials, RALES, was a double blind study in patients who had severe heart failure with left ventricular systolic dysfunction and were receiving standard therapy including ACE inhibitor treatment, a loop diuretic, and digoxin. Patients were randomly assigned to receive low dose MR antagonist, spironolactone or placebo added to their standard treatment. The trial was discontinued early due to an interim analysis showing the addition of spironolactone resulted in a 30% reduction in mortality and reducing SCD by 29%. In the next study, EPHESUS [Pitt et al. 2003] was designed to determine whether selective MR blockade with eplerenone could be tolerated by patients with acute myocardial infarction (AMI) complicated by heart failure due to systolic left ventricular dysfunction. Addition of the selective MR antagonist, eplerenone, substantially increased survival (15% reduction in mortality) and decreased hospitalization, and had a 21% reduction in SCD.

6. Conclusion

Since women do not present with severe left ventricular dysfunction and diagnosed CHD before SCD, they will not receive the current recommended treatment. Prospective studies are required that have the same proportion of women to men with ischemic heart disease to identify the sex-specific risk factors and pathophysiology of ischemic heart disease in women which leads to an adverse cardiovascular outcome [Malenka et al. 2002]. Further investigations are required to examine whether women will show the same benefit to adjunct treatment with angiotensin-converting enzyme (ACE) inhibitors, angiotensin receptor–blocking agents, lipid-lowering agents, mineralocorticoid receptor antagonists, thrombolytic and antithrombotic agents.

http://dx.doi.org/10.5772/55631

Author details

Anastasia Susie Mihailidou[1*], Rebecca Ritchie[2] and Anthony W. Ashton[3]

*Address all correspondence to: anastasia.mihailidou@sydney.edu.au

1 Department of Cardiology & Kolling Medical Research Institute Royal North Shore Hospital & University of Sydney, Sydney, Australia

2 Baker IDI Heart & Diabetes Institute, Melbourne, Australia

3 Perinatal Research Laboratories, Kolling Medical Research Institute Royal North Shore Hospital & University of Sydney, Sydney, Australia

References

[1] Zipes, D. P. Wellens HJJ ((1998). Sudden cardiac death. *Circulation. 98,* 2334-2351.

[2] Wong SH, Mulvihill NT, Norton M (2001). Assessing the risk of sudden cardiac death. *Heart.* 86: 624–625.

[3] Mazeika P (2001). Aborted sudden cardiac death: a clinical perspective. *Postgrad Med J.* 77: 363–370.

[4] Bairey Merz CN, Shaw LJ, Reis SE, et al ((2006). Insights from the NHLBI- Sponsored Women's Ischemia Syndrome Evaluation (WISE) Study. Part II: Gender differences in presentation, diagnosis, and outcome with regard to gender-based pathophysiology of atherosclerosis and macrovascular and microvascular coronary disease. *J Am Coll Cardiol.* 47(3): SS29., 21.

[5] Wake, R, Takeuchi, M, Yoshikawa, J, & Yoshiyama, M. (2007). Effects of gender on prognosis of patients with known or suspected coronary artery disease undergoing contrast-enhanced dobutamine stress echocardiography. *Circ J.* , 71(7), 1060-1066.

[6] Xhyheri, B, & Bugiardini, R. (2010). Diagnosis and Treatment of Heart Disease: Are Women Different From Men? *Progress in Cardiovascular Diseases.* , 53, 227-236.

[7] Melloni, C, Berger, J. S, Wang, T. Y, Gunes, F, Stebbins, A, Pieper, K. S, Dolor, R. J, Douglas, P. S, Mark, D. B, & Newby, L. K. (2010). Representation of women in randomized clinical trials of cardiovascular disease prevention. *Circ. Cardiovasc. Qual. Outcomes.* , 3, 135-142.

[8] Bell, D. M, & Nappi, J. (2000). Myocardial infarction in women: a critical appraisal of gender differences in outcomes. *Pharmacotherapy. 20,* 1034-1044.

[9] Mosca, L, Benjamin, E. J, Berra, K, Bezanson, J. L, Dolor, R. J, Lloyd-jones, D. M, Newby, L. K, Pina, I. L, Roger, V. L, Shaw, L. J, & Zhao, D. (2011). Effectiveness-

Based Guidelines for the Prevention of Cardiovascular Disease in Women-2011 Update. *Circulation.*, 123, 1243-1262.

[10] Priori, S. G, Aliot, E, Blomstrom-lundqvist, C, et al. (2001). Task Force on Sudden Cardiac Death of the European Society of Cardiology. *Eur Heart J. 22*, 1374-1450.

[11] Zheng, Z-J, Croft, J. B, Giles, W. H, et al. (2001). Sudden cardiac death in the United States, 1989 to 1998. *Circulation.*, 104, 2158-2163.

[12] Shaw, L. J, Merz, N. B, Pepine, C. J, Reis, S. E, Bittner, V, Kelsey, S. F, Olson, M, Johnson, B. D, Mankad, S, Sharaf, B. L, Rogers, W. J, Wessel, T. R, Arant, C. B, Pohost, G. M, Lerman, A, Quyyumi, A. A, & Sopko, G. for the WISE Investigators ((2006). Insights From the NHLBI-Sponsored Women's Ischemia Syndrome Evaluation (WISE) Study Part I: Gender Differences in Traditional and Novel Risk Factors, Symptom Evaluation, and Gender-Optimized Diagnostic Strategies. *J Am Coll Cardiol.* 47:4S-20S.

[13] Canto, J. G, Rogers, W. J, Goldberg, R. J, Peterson, E. D, Wenger, N. K, Vaccarino, V, Kiefe, C. I, Frederick, P. D, & Sopko, G. Zheng Z-J for the NRMI Investigators ((2012). Association of age and sex with myocardial infarction symptom presentation and In-Hospital mortality. *JAMA. 307*(8), 813-822.

[14] De Vreede-swagemakers, J. J, Gorgels, A. P, Dubois-arbouw, W. I, et al. (1997). Out-of-hospital cardiac arrest in the 19900s: a population-based study in the Maastricht area on incidence, characteristics and survival. *J Am Coll Cardiol.*, 30, 1500-1505.

[15] Kannel, W. B. Wilson PWF, D'Agostino RB, Cobb J ((1998). Sudden coronary death in women. *Am Heart J.*, 136, 205-212.

[16] Albert, C. M, Chae, C. U, Grodstein, F, Rose, L. M, Rexrode, K. M, Ruskin, J. N, Stampfer, M. J, & Manson, J. E. (2003). Prospective Study of Sudden Cardiac Death Among Women in the United States. *Circulation* , 107, 2096-2101.

[17] Dahlberg, S. T. (1990). Gender differences in risk factors for Sudden Cardiac Death. *Cardiology*. 77 (suppl 2): 31-40.

[18] Kim, C, Fahrenbruch, C. E, Cobb, L. A, et al. (2001). Out-of-hospital cardiac arrest in men and women. *Circulation* , 104, 2699-2703.

[19] Roger, V. L, Go, A. S, Lloyd-jones, D. M, Benjamin, E. J, Berry, J. D, Borden, W. B, Bravata, D. M, Dai, S, Ford, E. S, Fox, C. S, Fullerton, H. J, Gillespie, C, Hailpern, S. M, Heit, J. A, Howard, V. J, Kissela, B. M, Kittner, S. J, Lackland, D. T, Lichtman, J. H, Lisabeth, L. D, Makuc, D. M, Marcus, G. M, Marelli, A, Matchar, D. B, Moy, C. S, Mozaffarian, D, Mussolino, M. E, Nichol, G, Paynter, N. P, Soliman, E. Z, Sorlie, P. D, Sotoodehnia, N, Turan, T. N, Virani, S. S, Wong, N. D, Woo, D, & Turner, M. B. (2012). Heart Disease and Stroke Statistics-2012 Update A Report From the American Heart Association. *Circulation*. 125: ee230., 12.

[20] Lane, R. E, Cowie, M. R, & Chow, A. W. (2005). Prediction and prevention of sudden cardiac death in heart failure. *Heart* 2005;, 91, 674-680.

[21] Singh, S. N, Carson, P. E, & Fisher, S. G. (1997). Non-sustained ventricular tachycardia in severe heart failure. *Circulation.* , 96, 3794-3795.

[22] Kannel, W. B, & Schatzkin, A. (1985). Sudden death: lessons from subsets in population studies. *J Am Coll Cardiol.* 5: 141B-149B.

[23] Jouven, X, Desnos, M, Guerot, C, & Ducimetiere, P. (1999). Predicting sudden death in the population: the Paris Prospective Study I. *Circulation. 99*, 1978-1983.

[24] Khot, U. M, Khot, M. B, Bajzer, C. T, Sapp, S. K, Ohman, E. M, Brener, S. J, Ellis, S. G, Lincoff, A. M, & Topol, E. J. (2003). Prevalence of conventional risk factorsin patients with coronary heart disease.*JAMA* , 290, 898-904.

[25] Sandhu, R. K, Jimenez, M. C, Chiuve, S. E, Fitzgerald, K. C, Kenfield, S. A, Tedrow, U. B, & Albert, C. M. (2012). Smoking, smoking cessation, and risk of sudden cardiac death in women" *Circ Arrhythm Electrophysiol.* DOI:CIRCEP.112.975219.

[26] Schatzkln, A, Cupples, L. A, Heeren, T, Morelock, S, & Kannel, W. B. (1984). Sudden death in the Framlngham Heart Study: differences in Incidence and risk factors by sex and coronary disease status. *Am J Epidemiol. 120*, 888-899.

[27] Akiyama, T, Pawitan, Y, Greenberg, H, Kuo, C. S, & Reynolds-haertle, R. A. (1991). Increased risk of death and cardiac arrest from encainide and flecainide in patients after non-Q-wave acute myocardial infarction in the Cardiac Arrhythmia Suppression Trial: CAST Investigators. *Am J Cardiol. 68*, 1551-1555.

[28] Marsh, J. D, Lehmann, M. H, Ritchie, R. H, Gwathmey, J. K, Green, G. E, & Schiebinger, R. J. (1999). Androgen receptors mediate hypertrophy in cardiac myocytes. *Circulation.* , 98, 256-261.

[29] Paoletti, R, Cosignani, P. G, Kenemans, P, et al. (1997). Menopause: problems and interventions in the United States. In: Paoletti R, Cosignani PG, Kenemans P, Samsoe G, Soma M, Jackson AS, editors. Women's Health and Menopause. Norwell, MA: Kluwer Academic Publishers, , 9-14.

[30] Poehlman, E. T. (2002). Menopause, energy expenditure, and body composition. *Acta Obstet Gynecol Scand. 81*, 603-611.

[31] Lamon-fava, S. Wilson PWF, Schaefer EJ ((1996). Impact of body mass index on coronary heart disease risk factors in men and women: the Framingham Offspring study. *Arteriosler Thromb Vasc Biol.* 16L:, 1509-1515.

[32] Schierbeck, L. L, Rejnmark, L, Tofteng, C. L, Stilgren, L, Eiken, P, Mosekilde, L, Køber, L, & Jensen, J. E. (2012). Effect of hormone replacement therapy on cardiovascular events in recently postmenopausal women: randomised trial. BMJ. 2012 Oct 9; 345:e6409. doi:bmj.e6409.

[33] Huikuri, H. V, Castellanos, A, & Myerburg, R. J. Sudden death due to cardiac arrhythmias. *N Engl J Med.*, 345, 1473-1482.

[34] Orencia, A, Bailey, K, Yawn, B. P, & Kottke, T. E. (1993). Effect of gender on long-term outcome of angina pectoris and myocardial infarction/sudden unexpected death. *JAMA 269*, 2392-2397.

[35] Abildstrom, S. Z, Rask-madsen, C, Ottesen, M. M, Andersen, P. K, Rosthoj, S, Torp-pedersen, C, & Kober, L. (2002). Impact of age and sex on sudden cardiovascular death following myocardial infarction. *Heart.*, 88, 573-578.

[36] Adabag, A. S, Therneau, T. M, Gersh, B. J, Weston, S. A, & Roger, V. L. (2008). Sudden death after myocardial infarction. *JAMA.*, 300, 2022-2029.

[37] Verheugt, C. L, Uiterwaal, C. S, Van Der Velde, E. T, Meijboom, F. J, Pieper, P. G, Vliegen, H. W, Van Dijk, A. P, Bouma, B. J, Grobbee, D. E, & Mulder, B. J. (2008). Gender and outcome in adult congenital heart disease. *Circulation.*, 118, 26-32.

[38] Albert, C. M, Mcgovern, B. A, Newell, J. B, & Ruskin, J. N. (1996). Sex differences in cardiac arrest survivors. *Circulation.*, 93, 1170-1176.

[39] Chiuve, S. E, Fung, T. T, Rexrode, K. M, Spiegelman, D, Manson, J. E, Stampfer, M. J, & Albert, C. M. (2011). Adherence to a low-risk, healthy lifestyle and risk of Sudden Cardiac Death among women. *JAMA. 306*(1), 62-69.

[40] Albert, C. M, Nam, E. G, Rimm, E. B, Jin, H. W, Hajjar, R. J, & Hunter, D. J. MacRae CA, Ellinor PT ((2008). Cardiac Sodium Channel Gene Variants and Sudden Cardiac Death in Women. *Circulation.*, 117, 16-23.

[41] Nef, H. M, Möllmann, H, Akashi, Y. J, & Hamm, C. W. (2010). Mechanisms of stress (Takotsubo) cardiomyopathy. *Nat. Rev. Cardiol. 7*, 187-193.

[42] Abel, E. D, Litwin, S. E, & Sweeney, G. (2008). Cardiac remodeling in obesity. *Physiol Rev*, 88, 389-419.

[43] Anand, K, Mooss, A. N, & Mohiuddin, S. M. (2006). Aldosterone Inhibition Reduces the Risk of Sudden Cardiac Death in Patients with Heart Failure. *JRAAS. 7*, 15-19.

[44] Stecker, E. C, Vickers, C, Waltz, J, Socoteanu, C, John, B. T, Mariani, R, Mcanulty, J. H, Gunson, K, Jui, J, & Chugh, S. S. (2006). Population-based analysis of Sudden Cardiac Death with and without left ventricular systolic dysfunction. J Am Coll Cardiol., 47, 1161-1166.

[45] Chugh, S. S, Chung, K, Zheng, Z. J, John, B, & Titus, J. L. (2003). Cardiac pathologic findings reveal a high rate of sudden cardiac death of undetermined etiology in younger women. *Am Heart J.*, 146, 635-639.

[46] Beygui, F, Collet, J-P, Benoliel, J-J, Vignolles, N, Dumaine, R, Barthélémy, O, & Montalescot, G. (2006). High plasma aldosterone levels on admission are associated with

death in patients presenting with acute ST-elevation myocardial infarction. *Circulation.*, 114, 2604-2610.

[47] Palmer, B. R, Pilbrow, A. P, Frampton, C. M, et al. (2008). Plasma aldosterone levels during hospitalization are predictive of survival post-myocardial infarction. *Eur. Heart J.*, 29, 2489-2496.

[48] Tomaschitz, A, Pilz, S, Ritz, E, Meinitzer, A, Boehm, B. O, & Marz, W. (2010). Plasma aldosterone levels are associated with increased cardiovascular mortality: the Ludwigshafen Risk and Cardiovascular Health (LURIC) study. *Eur. Heart J. 31*, 1237-1247.

[49] Sheppard, K. E, & Autelitano, D. J. (2002). Beta-hydroxysteroid dehydrogenase 1 transforms 11-dehydrocorticosterone into transcriptionally active glucocorticoid in neonatal rat heart. *Endocrinology*, 143, 198-202.

[50] Gomez-sanchez, E. P, Venkataraman, M. T, Thwaites, D, & Fort, C. (1990). ICV infusion of corticosterone antagonizes ICV-aldosterone hypertension. *Am. J. Physiol.* 258: EE653., 649.

[51] Sato, A, & Funder, J. W. (1996). High glucose stimulates aldosterone-induced hypertrophy via type I mineralocorticoid receptors in neonatal rat cardiomyocytes. *Endocrinology 137*, 4145-4153.

[52] Young, M. J, & Funder, J. W. (1996). The renin-angiotensin-aldosterone system in experimental mineralocorticoid-salt-induced cardiac fibrosis. *Am. J. Physiol.* 271:EE888., 883.

[53] Makino, Y, Yoshikawa, N, Okamoto, K, Hirota, K, Yodoi, J, Makino, I, & Tanaka, H. (1999). Direct association with thioredoxin allows redox regulation of glucocorticoid receptor function. *J. Biol. Chem.*, 274, 3182-3188.

[54] Tamir, S, Izrael, S, & Vaya, J. (2002). The effect of oxidative stress on ERalpha and ERbeta expression. *J. Steroid Biochem. Mol. Biol.*, 81, 327-332.

[55] Zhang, Q, Piston, D. W, & Goodman, R. H. (2002). Regulation of corepressor function by nuclear NADH. *Science*, 295, 1895-1897.

[56] Fjeld, C. C, Birdsong, W. T, & Goodman, R. H. (2003). Differential binding of NAD+ and NADH allows the transcriptional corepressor carboxyl-terminal binding protein to serve as a metabolic sensor. *Proc. Natl. Acad. Sci. USA.*, 100, 9202-9207.

[57] Mihailidou, A. S. Le TYL, Mardini M, Funder JW ((2009). Glucocorticoids Activate Cardiac Mineralocorticoid Receptors During Experimental Myocardial Infarction. *Hypertension*, 54, 1306-1312.

[58] Ouvrard-pascaud, A, Sainte-marie, Y, Bénitah, J-P, et al. (2005). Conditional mineralocorticoid receptor expression in the heart leads to life-threatening arrhythmias. *Circulation.*, 11, 3025-3033.

[59] Mihailidou, AS, Bungaard, H, & Mardini, . (2000). Hyperaldosteronemia in rabbits inhibits the cardiac sarcolemmal Na +-K + pump. *Circ Res.* 86: 37-42.

[60] Mihailidou, A. S, Mardini, M, Funder, J. W, & Raison, M. (2002). Mineralocorticoid and Angiotensin Receptor Antagonism During Hyperaldosteronemia. *Hypertension.* , 40, 124-129.

[61] Tsuji, H. Venditti FJ Jr., Evans JC, Larson MG, Levy D ((1994). The associations of levels of serum potassium and magnesium with ventricular premature complexes (the Framingham Heart Study). *Am J Cardiol. 74,* 232-235.

[62] Stauffer, B. L, Sobus, R, & Sucharov, C. C. (2011). Sex differences in cardiomyocyte connexin43 expression. J Cardiovasc Pharmacol. 2011 July ; , 58(1), 32-39.

[63] Tribulova, N, Dupont, E, Soukup, T, Okruhlicova, L, & Severs, N. J. (2005). Sex differences in connexin-43 expression in left ventricles of aging rats. *Physiol Res.* , 54, 705-708.

[64] Knezl, V, Bacova, B, Kolenova, L, Mitasikova, M, Weismann, P, Drimal, J, & Tribulova, N. (2008). Distinct lethal arrhythmias susceptibility is associated with sex-related difference in myocardial connexin-43 expression. *Neuro Endocrinol Lett.* , 29, 798-801.

[65] Ai, J. Zhang R Li Y, Pu J, Lu Y, Jiao J, Li K, Yue B, Li Z, Wangg R, Wang L, Li Q, Wanga N, Shan N, Li Z, Yang B ((2010). Circulating microRNA-1 as a potential novel biomarker for acute myocardial infarction. *Biochem. Biophys. Res. Comm.* , 391, 73-77.

[66] Yang, B, Lin, H, Xiao, J, Lu, Y, Luo, X, Li, B, et al. (2007). The muscle-specific microRNA miR-1 regulates cardiac arrhythmogenic potential by targeting GJA1 and KCNJ2. *Nat. Med.* , 13, 486-491.

[67] Bardy, G. H, Lee, K. L, Mark, D. B, Poole, J. E, Packer, D. L, Boineau, R, Domanski, M, Troutman, C, Anderson, J, Johnson, G, Mcnulty, S. E, Clapp-channing, N, Davidson-ray, L. D, Fraulo, E. S, Fishbein, D. P, Luceri, R. M, & Ip, J. H. for the Sudden Cardiac Death in Heart Failure Trial (SCD-HeFT) Investigators ((2005). Amiodarone or an implantable cardioverter-defibrillator for congestive heart failure. N Engl J Med 2005;, 352, 225-37.

[68] Kadish, A, Dyer, A, Daubert, J. P, & Quigg, R. Estes NAM, Anderson KP, Calkins H, Hoch D, Goldberger J, Shalaby A, Sanders WE, Schaechter A, Levine JH, for the Defibrillators in Non-Ischemic Cardiomyopathy Treatment Evaluation (DEFINITE) Investigators ((2004). Prophylactic defibrillator implantation in patients with nonischemic dilated cardiomyopathy. *N Engl J Med.* , 350, 2151-2158.

[69] Wigginton, J. G, Pepe, P. E, Bedolla, J. P, Detamble, L. A, & Atkins, J. M. (2002). Sex related differences in the presentation and outcome of out-of-hospital cardiopulmonary arrest: A multiyear, prospective, population-based study. Crit Care Med. 30(Suppl 4):SS136., 131.

[70] DiMarco JP ((2003). Implantable cardioverter-defibrillators. *N Engl J Med.* , 349(19), 1836-1847.

[71] Pitt, B, Zannad, F, Remme, W. J, et al. (1999). The effect of spironolactone on morbidity and mortality in patients with severe heart failure: Randomized Aldactone Evaluation Study Investigators. *N Engl J Med.* , 341, 709-717.

[72] Pitt, B, Remme, W, Zannad, F, et al. (2003). Eplerenone Post-Acute Myocardial Infarction Heart Failure Efficacy and Survival Study Investigators. Eplerenone, a selective aldosterone blocker, in patients with left ventricular dysfunction after myocardial infarction. *N Engl J Med.* , 348, 1309-1321.

[73] Malenka, D. J, Wennberg, D. E, Quinton, H. A, et al. (2002). Gender-related changes in the practice and outcomes of percutaneous coronary interventions in northern New England 1994 to 1999. *J Am Coll Cardiol.* , 40, 2092-2101.

Chapter 5

Costs of Hospitalizations with a Primary Diagnosis of Acute Myocardial Infarction Among Patients Aged 18-64 Years in the United States

Guijing Wang, Zefeng Zhang, Carma Ayala,
Diane Dunet and Jing Fang

Additional information is available at the end of the chapter

http://dx.doi.org/10.5772/53499

1. Introduction

Acute Myocardial Infarction (AMI) is both a common and deadly type of cardiac event in the United States. Although the age-adjusted hospitalization rate for AMI and its in-hospital case fatality rates have both declined since the mid-1990s, there were still 634,000 inpatient admissions in 2009 for which AMI was listed as the primary diagnosis [1, 2]. Moreover, Americans suffered an estimated 610,000 first-time AMIs and 325,000 recurrent attacks, and 133,958 deaths in 2008 [2]. Because the declines in hospitalization and in-hospital mortality rates have been associated with more aggressive therapeutic interventions [1], it is important to evaluate the cost-effectiveness of these interventions.

To evaluate specifically the cost-effectiveness of various interventions against AMI, direct cost estimates of AMI are required [3-5]. Surprisingly, however, these cost estimates have not been comprehensively examined in the U.S. Many studies have investigated the economic burden of AMI, but all had some limitations [6-17]. Furthermore, in part because of limitations in available studies, the costs of coronary heart disease (CHD) were used in one study to represent the costs for AMI [6], albeit this is inappropriate. For example, a previous study of insured adults aged 18-64 years found that only about 30% of CHD cases represented AMI [9]. Moreover, the American Heart Association recently estimated that the total prevalence of CHD among persons aged ≥20 years was 7% but the AMI prevalence of AMI in this group was 3.1% [2]. In addition, in 2005, hospitalization costs for AMI admissions among adults aged 18-64 years were about $5000 more than those for CHD admissions of non-AMI [9]. Clearly, information on costs that does not clearly distinguish between AMI and non-AMI admissions is of little use in evaluating the cost-effectiveness of interventions to treat AMI [18].

In the present study we estimated AMI-specific costs by exploring the hospitalization costs of AMI while incorporating the impacts on costs of percutaneous coronary intervention (PCI), coronary artery bypass graft (CABG) surgery, comorbidities, complications, ST-elevation status, and length of stay (LOS) while controlling for age, sex, geographic regions, and urban versus non-urban location. Because PCI, CABG surgery, and LOS are likely to be the most influential factors on the costs and relevant factors for evaluating cost-effectiveness of AMI interventions, we also conducted multivariate logistic regressions to identify the factors predicting PCI, CABG surgery, and LOS.

2. Methods

2.1. Data source

The 2006-2008 MarketScan Commercial Claims and Encounter inpatient database was used for this study; this database contains information on patients up to age 64 years from approximately 40 privately insured employers, including state governments, with an average of nearly 21 million covered lives per year. In 2006-2008 the database had more than 2.4 billion service records representing commercially insured employees, qualified retirees and dependents from over 100 geographically diverse health insurance plans in all 50 U.S. states and the District of Columbia. The advantages of using the MarketScan database for economic studies include the large sample, detailed diagnosis codes for medical services, and hospitalization costs that are based on payment to providers [19]. Many researchers have used the MarketScan database to investigate medical costs associated with cardiovascular disease [9, 20, 21]

Using the International Classification of Diseases, 9th revision (ICD-9) codes, we identified hospitalizations with a primary diagnosis of AMI among patients aged 18-64 years who were enrolled in non-capitated health insurance plans. We further separated the hospitalizations into ST-elevated myocardial infarction (STEMI) and non-ST-elevated myocardial infarction (NSTEMI) cases. Based on secondary diagnosis codes, we identified major comorbidities, complications, and procedures for these hospitalizations (Table 1).

We excluded patients younger than 18 years because AMI is very uncommon in that group. We did not include patients in capitated health insurance plans because their costs of hospitalization would not reflect the medical services provided to them. We excluded hospitalizations with a LOS greater than 30 days because we determined that these hospitalizations (n=131, figure 1) would skew our results. To further limit the influence of extreme values on the cost estimates, we excluded all hospitalizations with a cost in the lowest or highest 1% of values (Figure 1). The costs in our study included all those for physician services, diagnostic tests, therapeutics, supplies, and room fees during the hospitalizations. These costs, as noted above, represented total payment to providers rather than hospital charges. Accordingly, we did not need to adjust charges into payments to reflect the true economic burden of hospitalizations, nor did we use unit cost per bed day or an expert panel's suggested cost as in many other studies [5, 11, 7, 22, 23]. We expressed the costs in 2008 dollars by adjusting the 2006 and 2007 value by the consumer price index (CPI) provided by the Bureau of Labor Statistics [24].

http://dx.doi.org/10.5772/53499

AMI, comorbidity, complication, or procedure	ICD-9 or CPT-4 code
AMI STEMI NSTEMI	410.xx 410.01, 410.11. 410.21. 410.31 410.71
Congestive heart failure	402.01, 402.11, 402.91, 404.01, 404.03,404.11, 404.13, 404.91, 404.93,428.xx
Hypertension	401.xx-405.xx
Diabetes	250.xx
Hyperlipidemia	272.xx
Kidney disease	403.xx, 404.xx, 582.xx, 583.xx, 585.xx, 586.xx, 587.xx
Stroke	430.xx-438.xx
Cardiogenic shock	785.51
Ventricular tachycardia	427.1
Ventricular fibrillation	427.41, 427.42
Atrial tachycardia	427.0
Atrial fibrillation	427.31, 427.32
PCI	92980-92982, 92984, 92995, 92996, 00.66, 36.01-36.09
CABG surgery	33510-33519, 33521-33523, 33533-33536, 36.10-36.19

AMI: Acute myocardial infarction.

ICD-9: International classification of disease, 9th revision.

CPT-4: Current procedural terminology, 4th revision.

STEMI: ST-elevated myocardial infarction.

NSTEMI: Non-ST-elevated myocardial infarction.

PCI: Percutaneous coronary intervention.

CABG: Coronary artery bypass graft.

Table 1. Diagnostic codes for acute myocardial infarction (AMI) and selected comorbidities and procedures

2.2. Statistical analysis

After deriving the sample means of the costs for different population groups, AMI types, comorbidities, complications, and procedures, we specified various versions of multivariate regression models to examine the factors influencing the costs while controlling for demographic variables and Charlson comorbidity index (CCI) [25]. We used CCI as a comprehensive measure of disease severity. It measures the likelihood of death or serious disability in the subsequent year by diagnosis codes of up to 18 different diseases. In addition to estimating the various versions of regression for the whole study sample, we ran a regression on the costs for STEMI and NSTEMI patients separately. Because PCI, CABG surgery and LOS were major factors determining the costs, we used logistic regression to investigate the predictors of these three factors. For the regression estimation, we used mixed-effects models with a repeated measures approach to account for the fact that a single patient might have multiple admissions during the 3-year period. All tests of statistical significance were 2-tailed, and a $p<0.001$ was considered significant. All statistical analyses were performed using SAS version 9.1 [26].

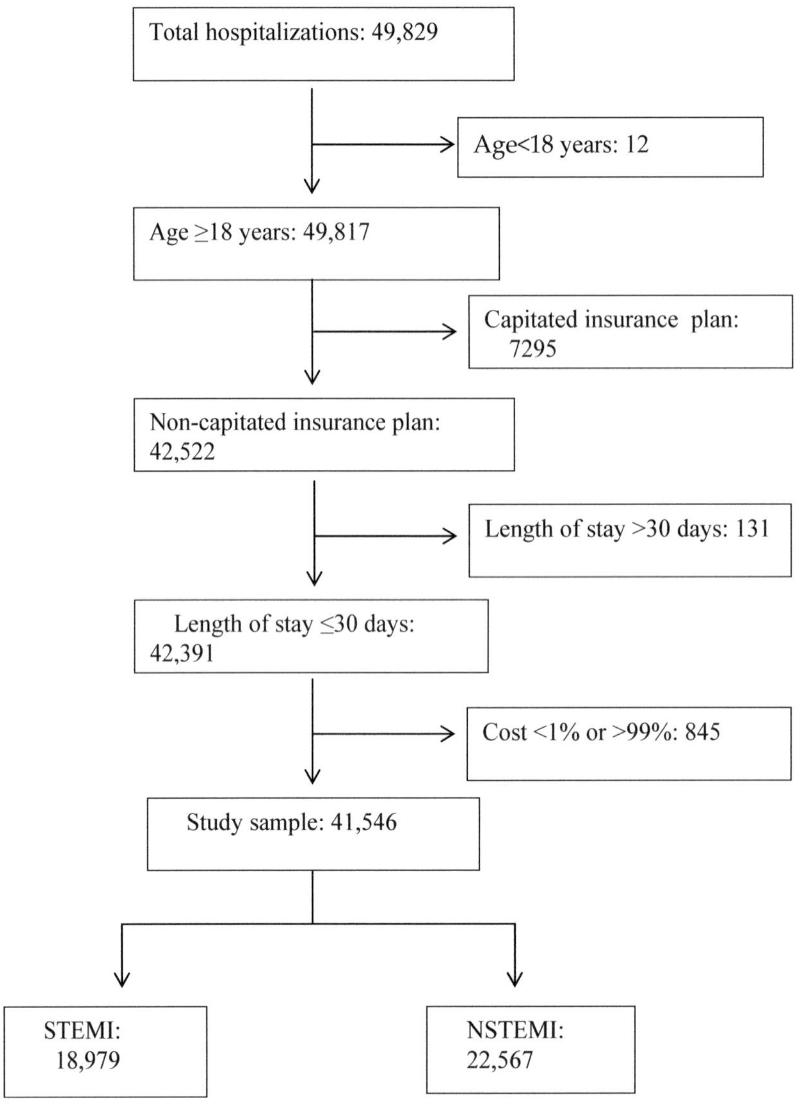

Figure 1. Diagram showing how the study sample was selected from all patients with a primary diagnosis of AMI in the 2006-2008 MarketScan Commercial Claims and Encounters inpatient database. STEMI: ST-elevated myocardial infarction. NSTEMI: non-ST-elevated myocardial infarction.

http://dx.doi.org/10.5772/53499

		N	Mean costs (± SD)
Total sample		41,546	29,840.2 ± 22,900.6
Age group (year)			
	18-44	4671	27,537.1 ± 20,693.3
	45-54	13,991	29,661.7 ± 22,073.7
	55-64	22,884	30,419.4 ± 23,778.6
Sex			
	Female	10,874	27,102.7 ± 22,110.1
	Male	30,672	30,810.7 ± 23,096.9
MSA			
	Yes	31,511	29,639.3 ± 22,661.9
	No	10,035	30,471.0 ± 23,624.5
Region			
	Northeast	3296	27,623.5 ± 22,012.1
	North Central	13,051	29,452.9 ± 21,927.1
	South	20,992	29, 637.4 ± 23,020.8
	West	4207	33,790.2 ± 25,373.3
AMI type			
	STEMI	18,979	32,030.3 ± 22,282.8
	NSTEMI	22,567	27,998.3 ± 23,248.8
Hypertension			
	Yes	16,020	29,403.5 ± 21,868.0
	No	25,526	30,114.3 ± 23,521.8
Congestive Heart Failure			
	Yes	4813	36,758.5 ± 29,163.4
	No	36,733	28,933.7 ± 21,786.3
Cancer			
	Yes	551	29,024.5 ± 23,356.1
	No	40,995	29,851.2 ± 22,894.5
Hyperlipidemia			
	Yes	14,075	29,375.3 ± 20,655.4
	No	27,471	30,078.4 ± 23,966.5
Peripheral vascular disease			
	Yes	296	34,324.6 ± 26,393.2

		N	Mean costs (± SD)
	No	41,250	29,808.0 ± 22,870.8
Diabetes			
	Yes	7367	31,917.7 ± 24,735.0
	No	34,179	29,392.4 ± 22,460.8
Obesity			
	Yes	2944	28,862.3 ± 21,845.5
	No	38,602	29,914.8 ± 22,977.6
Stroke			
	Yes	1739	42,133.5 ± 30,090.3
	No	39,807	29,303.2 ± 22,381.4
Kidney disease			
	Yes	1584	33,499.2 ± 27,595.5
	No	39,962	29,695.2 ± 22,682.8
PCI			
	Yes	27,062	30,960.8 ± 19,564.6
	No	14,484	27,746.5 ± 27,972.1
CABG			
	Yes	3879	63,105.9 ± 26,886.0
	No	37,667	26,414.5 ± 19,450.5
Cardiogenic shock			
	Yes	1135	53,016.1 ± 32,754.6
	No	40,411	29,189.3 ± 22,216.0
Ventricular tachycardia			
	Yes	2170	37,306.5 ± 27,619.9
	No	39,376	29,428.7 ± 22,540.5
Atrial tachycardia			
	Yes	299	29,365.2 ± 25,149.5
	No	41,247	29,843.6 ± 22,883.8
Ventricular fibrillation			
	Yes	1286	43,165.1 ± 29,468.8
	No	40,260	29,414.6 ± 22,530.4
Atrial fibrillation			
	Yes	1975	38,109.7 ± 28,974.3

http://dx.doi.org/10.5772/53499

	N	Mean costs (± SD)
No	39,571	29,427.5 ± 22,475.5
Charlson comorbidity index	41,456	1.55 ± 1.39
Length of stay (days)	41,456	4.66 ± 3.16

MSA: Metropolitan statistical area (resided in).

AMI: Acute myocardial infarction.

STEMI: ST-elevated myocardial infarction.

NSTEMI: Non-ST-elevated myocardial infarction.

PCI: Percutaneous coronary intervention.

CABG: Coronary artery bypass graft.

Table 2. Sample characteristics and mean costs (ages 18-64 years), 2006-2008 MarketScan inpatient database

3. Results

During 2006-2008, there were 41,546 hospitalizations with a primary diagnosis of AMI; their mean cost was $29,840 (± 22,901) (Table 2). Mean cost increased with age, but just marginally. Male patients cost more than female patients ($30,811 vs. $27,103, p<0.001), and the cost of STEMI exceeded that of NSTEMI ($32,030 vs. 27,998, p<0.001). Major comorbidities that increased the cost were stroke, heart failure, peripheral vascular disease, kidney disease, and diabetes. All of the complications except atrial tachycardia increased the cost greatly. Hospitalizations in which CABG surgery was performed cost a mean of $63,106, more than twice as high as the mean of $26,415 for those without CABG surgery. PCI increased the cost marginally.

The regression results indicated that age influenced the cost marginally after controlling for procedures, comorbidities, complications, LOS, and ST-elevation status, as well as other demographic variables (Model 6, Table 3). Hospitalizations of male patients had about $3350-$4000 higher costs than those of their female counterparts in Model 1-4, but the differences by sex dropped to $1437 when all the procedures and complications were considered (Model 6). The cost in the West was $5608 to $6530 higher than in any other regions in the fully adjusted model. The cost of hospitalization for STEMI was higher than that for NSTEMI, but the difference decreased from about $3776 (model 2) to $1003 with adjustment for all of the comorbidities, LOS, procedures, and complication (Model 6). CCI increased the cost by $2362 (Model 3), but this increase largely disappeared after adding the LOS, procedures, and complications (Model 6). Longer LOS increased the cost by about $2941 (p<0.001) per day (Model 6). After controlling for all other factors, PCI increased the cost by about $12,546, and CABG surgery increased the cost by about $28,406. These two procedures were the biggest factors influencing the cost of AMI hospitalizations. Complications increased the cost by $4669 in the fully adjusted model.

Independent variable	Model 1	Model 2	Model 3	Model 4	Model 5	Model 6	STEMI	NSTEMI
Age								
18-44 vs. 55-64	-2895.2 ±366.3 (<. 0001)	-3068.7 ±365.2 (<0.0001)	2278.4 ±362.4 (<0.0001)	64.9 ±307.7 (0.8329)	643.8 ±282.1 (0.0225)	808.3 ±281.0 (0.0040)	554.9 ± 420.3 (0.1868)	955.6 ±376.9 (0.0112)
45-54 vs. 55-64	-848.5 ±244.7 (0.0005)	-1024.1 ±244.13 (<0.0001)	564.5 ±242.1 (0.0197)	998.0 ±205.6 (<0.0001)	722.3 ±188.5 (0.0001)	817.3 ±187.8 (<0.0001)	502.8 ±283.7 (0.0763)	1069.4 ±249.6 (<0.0001)
Male	3720.4 ±254.5 (<0.0001)	3356.3 ±254.5 (<0.0001)	3804.2 ±252.4 (<0.0001)	3995.7 ±213.9 (<0.0001)	1574.6 ±198.0 (<0.0001)	1437.1 ±197.3 (<0.0001)	1046.8 ±316.9 (<0.0001)	1428.8 ±250.0 (<0.0001)
MSA	-829.5 ±262.0 (0.0015)	-834.6 ±261.1 (0.0014)	-805.1 ±258.5 (0.0018)	-1060.3 ±219.0 (<0.0001)	-1224.5 ±201.0 (<0.0001)	-1213.0 ±200.1 (<0.0001)	-1495.5 ±306.2 (<0.0001)	-903.1 ±263.2 (0.0006)
Region								
Northeast vs. West	-6009.0 ± 530.3 (<0.0001)	-5843.0 ±528.6 (<0.0001)	-6190.7 ±523.4 (<0.0001)	-7760.0 ±443.7 (<0.0001)	-6469.4 ±406.9 (<0.0001)	-6529.9 ±405.2 (<0.0001)	-7584.1 ±603.2 (<0.0001)	-5640.7 ± 546.4 (<0.0001)
North Central vs. West	-4235.0 ±404.0 (<0.0001)	-4045.4 ±402.8 (<0.0001)	-4349.7 ±398.8 (<0.0001)	-5570.7 ±338.1 (<0.0001)	-5693.6 ±309.9 (<0.0001)	-5735.1 ±308.6 (<0.0001)	-5444.2 ±454.0 (<0.0001)	-5894.0 ±420.8 (<0.0001)
South vs. West	-3980.0 ±385.3 (<0.0001)	-3771.9 ±384.2 (<0.0001)	-4291.2 ±380.7 (<0.0001)	-5985.3 ±322.9 (<0.0001)	-5561.9 ±296.0 (<0.0001)	-5608.2 ±294.8 (<0.0001)	-5959.2 ±431.8 (<0.0001)	-5266.7 ±403.3 (<0.0001)
STEMI	---	3775.6 ±224.8 (<0.0001)	4116.3 ±222.8 (<0.0001)	3654.9 ±188.9 (<0.0001)	1335.6 ±182.3 (<0.0001)	1002.8 ±182.4 (<0.0001)	---	---
Charlson comorbidity index	---	---	2361.8 ±80.3 (<0.0001)	-257.9 ±71.0 (0.0003)	169.1 ±65.3 (0.0085)	169.7 ±65.0 (0.0091)	361.6 ±11067 (0.0011)	80.9 ±79.5 (0.3091)
Length of stay	---	---	---	3974.8 ±31.1 (<0.0001)	3044.0 ±32.3 (<0.0001)	2940.7 ±32.6 (<0.0001)	3061.7 ±51.6 (<0.0001)	2865.5 ± 41.8 (<0.0001)
PCI	---	---	---	---	12490.0 ±204.5 (<0.0001)	12546.1 ±203.7 (<0.0001)	10169.0 ±366.5 (<0.0001)	13657.1 ±241.1 (<0.0001)

http://dx.doi.org/10.5772/53499

CABG	---	---	---	---	28189.4 ±352.7 (<0.0001)	28405.6 ±351.5 (<0.0001)	26476.2 ±599.8 (<0.0001)	29395.9 ±431.8 (<0.0001)
Complications	---	---	---	---	---	4669.1 ±252.5 (<0.0001)	4803.8 ±350.6 (<0.0001)	4498.8 ±368.0 (<0.0001)

Model 1: Age, sex, MSA, and region;

Model 2: Model 1 + STEMI;

Model 3: Model 2 + comorbidities;

Model 4: Model 3 + length of stay;

Model 5: Model 4 + PCI, CABG surgery;

Model 6: Model 5 + complications;

MSA: Metropolitan statistical area (resided in).

STEMI: ST-elevated myocardial infarction.

NSTEMI: Non-ST-elevated myocardial infarction.

PCI: Percutaneous coronary intervention.

CABG: Coronary artery bypass graft.

Table 3. Coefficient estimates of hospitalization costs for patients with acute myocardial infarction

PCI and CABG surgery increased the cost for both the STEMI and NSTEMI groups, with both procedures increasing the cost more for the NSTEMI group than for STEMI. LOS, in contrast, increased the cost more for the STEMI than the NSTEMI group, while living in an urban area (MSA in Table 3) decreased cost by $1496 for STEMI and $903 for NSTEMI.

Logistic regression indicated that patients aged 18-44 years were less likely than those aged 55-64 to undergo PCI or to have CABG surgery, and they were more likely to have a shorter LOS (i.e., <5 days) (Table 4). Patients in urban area were more likely to have PCI, but less likely to have CABG. Men were more likely to undergo PCI or to have CABG surgery than were women, but their odd of a short LOS was greater. Versus patients who did not live in urban areas, urban patients were more likely to have PCI, but they were less likely to undergo CABG surgery. Compared with patients in the West, patients in other regions were more likely to have a long LOS (i.e., ≥5 days), but they were usually less likely to have PCI and CABG surgery, with PCI in the North Central region the exception. STEMI patients were more likely than NSTEMI patients to undergo PCI and CABG surgery, and they were more likely to have a long LOS. Patients with comorbidities or complications were more likely to have a long LOS, but they were less likely to have PCI or CABG surgery. Patients undergoing PCI were more likely to have a short LOS, while patients undergoing CABG surgery were far more likely to have a long LOS.

Independent variable	PCI (yes vs. no)	CABG (yes vs. no)	Length of stay (<5 vs. ≥5)
Age 18-44 vs. 55-64 years	0.877 (0.814, 0.944)	0.718 (0.616, 0.836)	0.706 (0.651, 0.765)
Age 45-54 vs. 55-64 years	1.170 (1.112, 1.232)	1.010 (0.921, 1.107)	0.807 (0.767, 0.851)
Male	1.813 (1.724, 1.907)	2.776 (2.502, 3.081)	0.760 (0.721, 0.801)
MSA	1.249 (1.184, 1.317)	0.905 (0.824, 0.995)	1.044 (0.988, 1.104)
Region			
Northeast vs. West	0.792 (0.711, 0.884)	0.488 (0.391, 0.608)	1.560 (1.392, 1.747)
North Central vs. West	1.153 (1.059, 1.256)	0.969 (0.830, 1.132)	1.267 (1.158, 1.387)
South vs. West	0.884 (0.815, 0.959)	0.934 (0.806, 1.081)	1.486 (1.364, 1.620)
STEMI vs. NSTEMI	4.514 (4.293, 4.746)	1.337 (1.219, 1.467)	1.333 (1.267, 1.402)
Charlson comorbidity index	0.890 (0.876, 0.905)	0.887 (0.862, 0.913)	1.432 (1.408, 1.457)
Length of stay (days)	0.981 (0.973, 0.990)	1.405 (1.388, 1.422)	---
PCI	---	0.060 (0.053, 0.067)	0.819 (0.776, 0.866)
CABG	0.062 (0.056, 0.069)	---	47.992 (41.288, 55.785)
Complications	0.894 (0.834, 0.959)	0.863 (0.771, 0.966)	2.621 (2.460, 2.793)

PCI: Percutaneous coronary intervention.

CABG: Coronary artery bypass graft.

MSA: Metropolitan statistical area (resided in).

STEMI: ST-elevated myocardial infarction.

NSTEMI: Non-ST-elevated myocardial infarction.

Table 4. Coefficient estimates of logistic regression of PCI, CABG, and length of stay

4. Discussion

The large number of hospitalizations in our economic study of inpatients who had suffered an AMI enabled us to explore a variety of factors that influenced their costs. The results suggest that CABG and PCI are the biggest drivers of hospital costs for AMI patients, adding, respectively, $12,546 and $28,406 to the cost of a stay. The cost effects of PCI and CABG in our study were comparable to the $15,089 and $28,974 additional costs, respectively, found in a Medicare population [7]. Another study reported similar costs for PCI and CABG [17]. In an earlier study using MarketScan data from 2003 to 2006, Zhao and Winget found that the total hospitalization costs of PCI and CABG surgery patient costs were, respectively,

$31,379 and $63,909 [10]. Unfortunately, Zhao and Winget did not explore the effects of PCI and CABG on the costs of stay, as we did in our study. Such information is needed to evaluate the cost-effectiveness of AMI interventions [4].

Two other significant drivers of cost in our study were complications and LOS. Having one or more complications increased the cost by over $4600, and LOS increased the cost by over $2900 per day. LOS was highly correlated with CABG surgery and with complications, as indicated in our logistic models (Table 4). Thus, interventions aiming to prevent or better manage the complications of AMI patients might be cost-effective in reducing the hospitalization costs of this group.

Hospitalizations with STEMI had, on average, higher costs than NSTEMI hospitalizations, but after including PCI and CABG surgery as well as complications, comorbidities, and LOS in the regression model, the magnitude of the effect became much smaller. This may be because of differences in treatment approaches and in complications between the two kinds of hospitalizations. For example, over 80% of STEMI hospitalizations had a PCI while only about 51% in the NSTEMI group did. However, the NSTEMI group had a higher rate of CABG surgery than did STEMI (12% vs. 8%) (not shown in tables). On the other hand, compared with NSTEMI cases, the STEMI group had a higher rate of cardiogenic shock, ventricular tachycardia, and ventricular fibrillation, but it had a lower rate of heart failure, atrial tachycardia, and atrial fibrillation. All of these factors would affect the cost differences between STEMI and NSTEMI hospitalizations. The fact that STEMI cost more than NSTEMI was consistent with the literature; in Mexico, for example, STEMI cost nearly $2800 more than NSTEMI [11].

The predictors of PCI, CABG surgery, and LOS that we set forward in this study provide important information for secondary cost-effectiveness analyses of AMI interventions. We found that male patients were more likely than females to have PCI and CABG surgery, but their odds of a shorter LOS (<5 days) were greater. STEMI status greatly increased the probability of having PCI (coefficient estimate of 4.514) and significantly increased the probability of CABG surgery (coefficient estimate of 1.337), and it was associated with greater odds of a longer LOS (≥5 days). Patients with comorbidities and complications were relatively less likely to undergo PCI and CABG surgery, but they were more likely to have a longer LOS. All of these results could be used as inputs in cost-effectiveness evaluations of AMI interventions.

The numerous strengths of this study notwithstanding, several limitations should be considered when interpreting our results. First, all of our patients were covered by non-capitated private insurance plans. Although the costs of these patients accurately reflect the true economic burden imposed by their hospitalizations, the special population may have limited the generalizability of our results to the broader U.S. population. Second, all of our patients were 18-64 years old. The elderly population (aged >64 years) has much higher incidence and prevalence of AMI and its related comorbidities and complications [1, 2]; as a consequence, the total costs of AMI should be higher in this population than among those 18-64. Although many studies have focused on the cost of AMI among the elderly [4, 5, 8], new estimation methods are needed along with high-quality data to develop better cost estimates for this population. Unfortunately, our data would not be appropriate for an analysis of costs among the elderly population for AMI hospitalization. A third limitation is that we estimated the costs of hospitalizations only. With survival rates increasing because of advances in technology [1], AMI patients are living longer. Correspondingly, the lifetime costs of outpatient care and medications for afflicted patients should be increasing. Additionally, productivity losses from the morbidity and premature mortality associated with AMI are also high [10] and should be considered in any comprehensive economic evaluations.

Given all of these factors, the hospitalization costs presented in our report should be treated as a conservative estimate of the economic burden associated with AMI. Moreover, we should note the limitation that we analyzed the costs of hospitalizations with AMI as a *primary* diagnosis. Although this decision let us cover the majority of AMI cases, there may be substantial additional hospitalizations in which AMI is a secondary diagnosis [9]. These hospitalizations should certainly be included in any complete analysis of the costs of hospitalizations of AMI patients. Because examining the costs of AMI as a secondary diagnosis would require a different analytical framework from the one we used, it would have been beyond the scope of our analysis.

5. Conclusion

Using a large set of claims data, we estimated the hospitalization costs of patients with a primary diagnosis of AMI and identified the main cost drivers of this important problem. Because most previous studies did not provide any information on the predictors of the costs of AMI hospitalizations [27], we hope that the present study has to some degree filled this gap in the literature. The high costs of AMI could be an economic justification for policy makers to support efforts to prevent AMI. In addition, the detailed information presented herein about the impact of various factors on the costs, procedures, and LOS associated with hospitalizations having a primary diagnosis of AMI can be used to evaluate and support health economic research such as studies on the cost-effectiveness of interventions to control this problem.

Author details

Guijing Wang*, Zefeng Zhang, Carma Ayala, Diane Dunet and Jing Fang

*Address all correspondence to: Gbw9@cdc.gov

Division for Heart Disease and Stroke Prevention, Centers for Disease Control and Prevention (CDC), Atlanta, GA, USA

The findings and conclusions of this article are those of the authors and do not necessarily represent the official position of the US Centers for Disease Control and Prevention (CDC).

References

[1] Fang J, Alderman MH, Keenan NL, Ayala C. Acute myocardial infarction hospitalization in the United States, 1979 to 2005. Am J Med 2010; 123: 259-66.

[2] American Heart Association. Heart disease and stroke statistics – 2012 update: a report from the American Heart Association. Circulation 2012; 125: e2-e220.

[3] Ioannides-Demos LL, Makarounas-Kirchmann K, Ashton E, Stoelwinder J, McNeil JJ. Cost of myocardial infarction to the Australian community: a prospective, mutlticentre survey. Clin Drug Investig 2010; 30: 533-43.

[4] Sloss EM, Wickstrom SL, McCaffrey DF, et al. Direct medical costs attributable to acute myocardial infarction and ischemic stroke in cohorts with atherosclerotic conditions. Cerebrovasc Dis 2004; 18: 8-15.

[5] Krumholz HM, Chen J, Murillo JE, Cohen DJ, Radford MJ. Clinical correlates of in-hospital costs for acute myocardial infarction in patients 65 years of age and older. Am Heart J 1998; 135: 523-31.

[6] Turpie AG. Burden of disease: medical and economic impact of acute coronary syndromes. Am J Manag Care 2006; 12: S430-4.

[7] Kugelmass AD, Cohen DJ, Brown PP, Simon AW, Becker ER, Culler SD. Hospital resources consumed in treating complications associated with percutaneous coronary interventions. Am J Cardiol 2006; 97: 322-7.

[8] Tiemann O. Variations in hospitalisation costs for acute myocardial infarction – a comparison across Europe. Health Econ 2008; 17: S33-45.

[9] Wang G, Zhang Z, Ayala C, Dunet D, Fang J. Inpatient costs associated with ischemic heart disease among adults aged 18-64 years in the United States. In: Lakshmanados U, Ed. Novel strategies in ischemic heart disease. Rijeka, Croatia: InTech 2012; pp. 319-32.

[10] Zhao Z, Winget M. Economic burden of illness of acute coronary syndromes: medical and productivity costs. BMC Health Serv Res 2011; 11: 35. http://www.biomedcentral.com/1472-6963/11/25.

[11] Reynales-Shigematsu LM, Campuzano-Rincon JC, Sesma-Vasquez S, et al. Costs of medical care for acute myocardial infarction attributable to tobacco consumption. Arch Med Res 2006; 37: 871-9.

[12] Eisenstein EL, Shaw LK, Anstrom KJ, et al. Assessing the clinical and economic burden of coronary artery disease: 1986-1998. Med Care 2001; 39: 824-35.

[13] Etemad LR, McCollam PL. Total first-year costs of acute coronary syndrome in a managed care setting. J Manag Care Pharm 2005; 11: 300-6.

[14] McCollam P, Etemad L. Cost of care for new-onset acute coronary syndrome patients who undergo coronary revascularization. J Invasive Cardiol 2005; 17: 307-11.

[15] Menzin J, Wygant G, Hauch O,Jackel J, Friedman M. One-year costs of ischemic heart disease among patients with acute coronary syndromes: findings from a multi-employer claims database. Curr Med Res Opin 2008; 24): 461-8.

[16] Russell MW, Huse DM, Drowns S, Hamel EC, Hartz SC. Direct medical costs of coronary artery disease in the United States. Am J Cardiol 1998; 81: 1110-5.

[17] Kauf TL, Velazquez EJ, Crosslin DR, et al. The cost of acute myocardial infarction in the new millennium: evidence from a multinational registry. Am Heart J 2006; 151: 206-12.

[18] Luengo-Fernandez R, Gray AM, Rothwell PM. Costs of stroke using patient-level data: a critical review of the literature. Stroke. 2009; 40: e18-23.

[19] Adamson DM, Chang S, Hansen LG. Health research data from the real world: the MarketScan database (white paper). 2008. Available from http://thomsonreuters.com. Requested May 2010.

[20] Wang G, Zhang Z, Ayala C. Hospitalization costs associated with hypertension as a secondary diagnosis among insured patients aged 18-64 years. Am J Hypertens 2010; 23: 275-81.

[21] Kahende JW, Woollery TA, Lee CW. Assessing medical expenditures on 4 smoking-related diseases, 1996-2001. Am J Health Behav 2007; 31: 601-11.

[22] Ringborg A, Yin DD, Martinel M, Stalhammar J, Linggren P. The impact of acute myocardial infarction and stroke on health care costs in patients with type 2 diabetes in Sweden. Eur J Cardiovasc Prev Rehabil 2009; 16: 576-82.

[23] Wang G, Dietz WH. Economic burden of obesity in youths aged 6 to 17 years: 1979-1999. Pediatrics 2002; 109: e81. http://www.pediatrics.org/cgi/content/full/109/5/e81.

[24] Bureau of Labor Statistics (BLS). Consumer price index (CPI). Available from ftp://ftp.bls.gov/pub/special.requests/cpi/cpiai.txt. Accessed March 16, 2012.

[25] Charlson ME, Pompei P, Ales KL, MacKenzie CR. A new method of classifying prognostic comorbidity in longitudinal studies: development and evaluation. J Chronic Dis 1987;40:373-383.

[26] SAS. SAS/STAT User's Guide. Cary NC: SAS Institute Inc.; 2007.

[27] Tarride JE, Lim M, DesMeules M, et al. A review of the cost of cardiovascular disease. Can J Cardiol 2009; 25: e195-202.

Chapter 6

Biomarkers of Cardiac Ischemia

David C. Gaze

Additional information is available at the end of the chapter

http://dx.doi.org/10.5772/55250

1. Introduction

Ischemia (from the Greek ισχαιμία, *ischaimía*; *isch-* root denoting a restriction or thinning or to make or grow thin, *haema* blood) is the restriction of blood supply and thus the inadequate delivery of oxygen and removal of carbon dioxide from cellular tissue. This imbalance may lead to dysfunctional or permanent damage to the affected tissue and organ.

Cardiac ischemia occurs when there is a supply versus demand mismatch in coronary blood flow. In patients who present with unstable angina, ischemia occurs due to partial or total occlusion of a coronary artery due to plaque rupture. In stable angina however, there is progressive vascular occlusion resulting ultimately in a luminal stenosis of greater than 70%, impeding blood flow to the distal tissue. If the ischemia is reversible, no permanent myocardial damage occurs.If however the ischemic episode is prolonged; there will be cellular necrosis which will lead to acute myocardial infarction (AMI).The immediate clinical challenge is to be able to identify acutely impaired myocardial perfusion before the necrotic process starts. Currently, the only strategy for this is to detect ST-segment changes on the electrocardiogram (ECG), however the ECG is non-diagnostic in many cases. The sensitivity of the admission ECG for the diagnosis of AMI is typically around 50%. Reperfusion, be it pharmacological or surgical, is the essential life-saving intervention with the aim of salvaging myocardial tissue localised at the affected site. Many patients however who present with chest pain to the emergency department (ED) do not have a final diagnosis of AMI. There is therefore a need for a strategy which could detect cardiac ischemia before necrosis occurs and result in prompt revascularisation. Blood borne biomarkers for ischemia may be of diagnostic and prognostic value.

To date, a number of candidate biomarkers of ischemia are being researched. However, one, Ischemia modified albumin (IMA®), has been developed into a commercially available cardiac biomarker assay and licensed for routine clinical application both by CE marking in Europe and Food and Drug Administration (FDA) approval in the United States. This chapter will explore the rational for the necessity of cardiac ischemia biomarker testing and detail the development of the IMA assay with emphasis on its clinical and prognostic utility.

1.1. The cardiovascular disease epidemic

Cardiovascular disease (CVD) accounts for the majority of global deaths. CVD was responsible for 29% of all global deaths in 2004. According to the World Heart Federation, CVD is responsible for 17.1 million deaths globally each year. Surprisingly, 82% of these deaths occur in the developing world. Such numbers are often difficult to comprehend. CVD is responsible for one in every five deaths disease kills one person every 34 seconds in the USA alone. 35 people under the age of 65 die prematurely in the United Kingdom every day due to CVD. It is predicted that by 2030 23 million people will die annually from a cardiovascular related disease. Data from the USA suggests that CVD was responsible for 34% of all deaths in 2006 and over 151,000 Americans who died were under 65 years of age.

1.2. Acute chest pain

Patients with chest pain constitute the largest single category of patients admitted to hospitals in the UK [1]. In the USA, registry data recorded 11.2 million chest pain presentations to the ED in 2008 alone. The presentations are also diagnostically challenging. The majority of admissions have either stable ischemic heart disease (IHD) or no ischemic heart disease [2]. Such admission episodes are often short and clinically inappropriate. Conversely, it has been estimated that between 2 and 7% of patients with AMI are inappropriately discharged from the ED [3, 4] and suffer disproportionate morbidity and mortality. Attempts to improve diagnosis have included risk scoring systems [5], computerised decision support [6, 7] and automated ECG interpretation [8]. Although clinical assessment remains integral to the assessment of patients with chest pain, cardiac biomarker measurement has become an essential component in the diagnostic armamentarium.

2. Pathophysiology of cardiac ischemia

The mechanisms involved in the development of cardiovascular disease are multifactorial and include abnormalities in cholesterol and lipid metabolism, inflammation and oxidative stress processes within the vascular wall, cellular disruption to the endothelium and intra-lumenal platelet activation/aggregation. The ischemia cascade from initiation of local ischemia to the development of symptomatic chest pain is depicted in figure 1.The pathological processes responsible for the development of atherosclerotic lesions and endothelial dysfunction are advanced far earlier than when patients typically become symptomatic and present with chest pain. The disease process does not occur in distinct episodes but rather is a continuum from asymptomatic vascular dysfunction thorough to angina in those with myocardial ischemia, which, without intervention can progress to non-ST segment elevation myocardial infarction (NSTEMI) or cumulate into ST segment elevation myocardial infarction (STEMI). Patients

http://dx.doi.org/10.5772/55250

presenting at any stage in the process may be diagnosed with acute coronary syndrome (ACS). The earlier in the disease continuum the presentation is; the greater the opportunity for successful myocardial tissue preservation. As there is no definitive biomarker for ischemia, current treatment focuses on the need for urgent therapeutic revascularisation in patients with established cardiac necrosis, identified by the cardiac troponins.

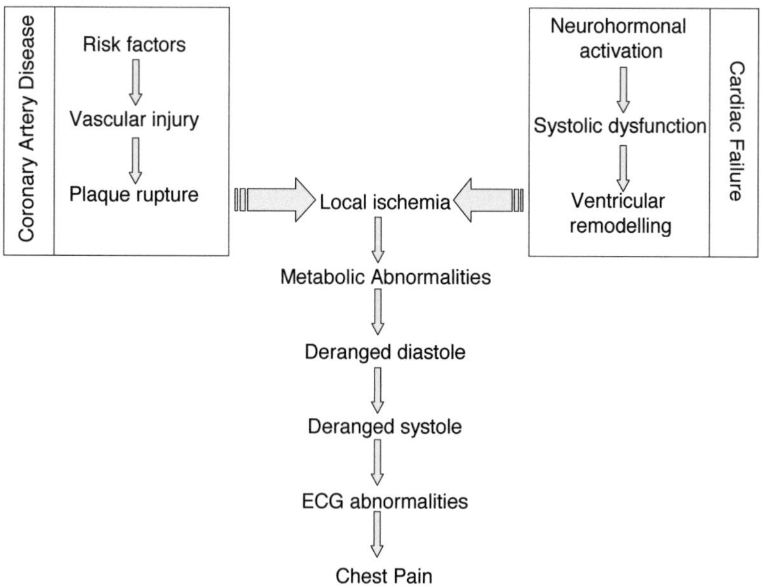

Figure 1. Development of Ischemia in the ischemia cascade.

The pathological process unless disrupted by therapeutic intervention results in the death of cardiac myocytes. Predisposing this terminal event, a vulnerable atherosclerotic plaque becomes disrupted exposing the thrombogenic lipid core and sub endothelium to the luminal milieu. Exposure results in platelet activation and aggregation and along with the coagulation cascade, an intracoronary thrombus forms. The thrombus may not obstruct the lumen and the patient is asymptomatic, however if the lumen is totally occluded, AMI will ensue. A partially occluded lumen and reduced oxygen supply both contribute to the development of ischemic myocardium.

3. Clinical detection of cardiac ischemia

The clinical presentation of cardiac ischemia is difficult to definitively diagnose. Currently there is no gold standard test to detect ischemia however a number of reliable tests exist.

Historically patients were admitted for monitoring or discharged on the basis of clinical interpretation by the ED physician. It is accepted that this is no longer acceptable clinical practice.

The typical presentation is exertional or stress induced central chest pain. These episodes usually last from a few minutes to hours and can resolve upon rest. Common descriptions by the patient include tightness, crushing stabbing or burning pain. Patients may also have nausea and vomiting, dyspnoea, palpitations. Typical symptoms increase the likelihood of an AMI however atypical presentations cannot be used to exclude AMI. Women, the elderly and those with diabetes mellitus often present with atypical chest pain.

The clinical history and physical examination will assess the presence of risk factors for AMI, however alone; the initial clinical examination is insensitive and unspecific for diagnosis. It may however give insight to differential or alternative diagnoses in those patients who, upon further investigation do not have an AMI. The 12 lead ECG is additive to the physical examination. The majority of ECG traces performed at admission are non-diagnostic with approximately 5% of suspected AMI patients having a diagnostic trace indicative of AMI. Although the ECG is relatively insensitive, the presence of ST segment elevation however is 100% diagnostic for AMI and serves as the criterion for immediate induction of fibrinolytic therapy or emergency interventional revascularization.

3.1. Cardiac imaging

Recently cardiac imaging has played an important role in the detection of ischemia. Perfusion abnormalities can be detected by single-photon emission computer tomography (SPECT) myocardial perfusion imaging (MPI) and mechanical dysfunction can be detected by echocardiography or gated MPI. Gated SPECT MPI can identify regional and global dysfunction of the left ventricle as ischemia impairs myocellular contractility. SPECT requires uptake of an isotope by active membrane transport mechanisms and caution should be advised in those patients with impaired renal clearance. Both echocardiography and SPECT are sensitive and specific and have a high negative predictive value for the diagnosis and prognosis of patients with suspected ACS. These diagnostic modalities however are grossly expensive, time consuming, technically more challenging and are not as widely available as compared to the simple ECG or a blood borne biomarker. The use cardiac imaging in the ED on a 24 hour, 7 day a week basis is therefore compromised.

3.2. Cardiac biomarkers of ischemia

There have been progressive developments within basic and clinical research to identify candidate biomarkers of ischemia and to develop simple to use assays. Any such assay needs to have similar analytical (limit of detection, precision, reference intervals) and clinical performance (sensitivity, specificity, risk stratification and predictive value) compared to that of markers of necrosis, such as high sensitivity cardiac troponin assays. A number of candidate biomarkers have been identified. However very few make it from a research grade assay to a fully licenced automated assay for clinical use. The most promising biomarkers to date are reviewed below. Of these, Ischemia Modified Albumin has been the most successful biomarker and greater attention is given to this marker.

4. Malondialdehyde low density lipoprotein

Malondialdehyde low density lipoprotein (MDA-LDL) is a sensitive biomarker for ACS patients with unstable angina and AMI. MDA is a candidate compound which causes oxidative modification of LDL. MDA (propanedial, $C_3H_4O_2$) is a reactive aldehyde produced by degradation of polyunsaturated lipids or released during prostanoid metabolism. This reactive oxygen species causes oxidative modification to LDL. MDA-LDL reacts with the charged amino group of B-100 protein lysyl residues. Plasma concentrations of MDA-LDL identify patients with coronary artery disease. Modified LDL may also instigate an immune response leading to autoantibody and LDL immune complex production. MDA-LDL not only serves as an oxidative stress marker but as a marker of plaque destabilisation.

5. Myeloperoxidase

Myeloperoxidase (MPO, EC 1.11.2.2, 1.11.2.2) is a 150 KDa protein dimer consisting of two 15 KDa light chains and two variable weight glycosylated heavy chains bound by a heme group responsible for the green colour when secreted in pus and mucus. There are three known isoforms which differ in the size of the heavy chain [9]. It is encoded by the MPO gene located on chromosome 17 [10]. MPO is most abundant in neutrophil granulocytes. It is a lysosomal enzyme stored in azurophilic granules of polymorphonucleocytes and macrophages. MPO catalyses the conversion of chloride and hydrogen peroxide into hypochlorite (hypochlorous acid). Furthermore, MPO oxidises tyrosine to the tyrosyl radical using hydrogen peroxide as an oxidising agent. Both hypochlorite and the tyrosyl radical are cytotoxic and are produce to kill pathogens in response to infection. Elevation in MPO is therefore not indicative of cardiac ischemia, as increases occur in infection, inflammation and infiltrative disease processes, thus reducing the specificity for cardiac ischemia.

MPO may contribute to the pathophysiology of ACS, as the hypochlorite end product is an oxidizing agent of low density lipoprotein (LDL) and may play a key role in the degradation of collagen and contributing to the destabilisation of the plaque. Patients with ACS who have elevated MPO are at risk of short and long-term adverse outcomes. In a case-control study from the USA, Zhang and colleagues demonstrate that MPO concentrations are significantly greater in patients (n=158) with coronary artery disease compared to controls (n=175) who do not demonstrate angiographically significant coronary disease [11]. Plasma MPO concentrations identify patients at risk of major adverse cardiac events in the absence of necrosis. In 604 sequential chest pain admissions, MPO predicted adverse cardiac events (AMI, need for revascularisation or death)at 30 days (odds ratio 2.2, 95%CI 1.1-4.6) and 6 months (odds ratio 4.1, 95%CI 2.0-8.4) [12].

6. Whole blood choline

Choline (2-hydroxy-N,N,N-trimethylethanaminium, $C_5H_{11}NO$) is a water soluble essential nutrient. It is a product of phosphodiesteric cleavage of membrane phospholipids such as phosphatidylcholine and sphingomyelin; catalysed by phospholipase D (EC 3.1.4.4). Choline is the precursor to actylcholine production.

Physiologically choline provides cell structural integrity, is the precursor for acetylcholine production and a source of methyl groups that participate in the S-adenosylmethionine synthesis pathway.

Whole blood (WBCHO) and plasma choline concentrations increase after stimulation of phospholipase D and the activation of coronary plaque cell surface receptors or ischemia. Phospholipase D activation in coronary plaques causes stimulation of macrophage by oxidised LDL, secretion of matrix metalloproteinase enzymes and activation of platelets. WBCHO can be measured by high performance liquid chromatography coupled to mass spectrometry (HPLC-MS). In a study of over 300 patients with suspected ACS, WBCHO measured at admission was a significant predictor of cardiac death, cardiac arrest, arrhythmia, heart failure or the need for percutaneous coronary intervention (PCI) at 30 day follow up [13]. The predictive power was enhanced by the addition of either cTnT or cTnI and served not as a marker of myocardial cell necrosis but identified patients at high risk with unstable angina. WBCHO is therefore a better predictive tool than plasma choline for early risk stratification in patients who are cardiac troponin negative on admission. The current detection methodology using HPLC-MS is not suitable for urgent clinical use.

7. Free fatty acids

Fatty acids are carboxylic acid molecules with a long aliphatic tail known as a chain, which are either saturated or unsaturated. Most naturally occurring fatty acids have an even number of carbon atoms (4 to 28) in the tail region. Fatty acids are produced from the breakdown of triglyceride or phospholipid. The majority fatty acids circulate bound to albumin with a very small percentage appearing as the unbound free fatty acid (FFAu) form [14]. The circulating level of FFA is limited to the availability of the albumin binding sites.

The mechanism of FFAu release is not fully understood however increased catecholamines following cardiac ischemia may activate FFAu release following lipolysis in adipocytes. FFAu are 14-fold higher post-PCI, compared to pre procedural concentrations and were higher in those with associated ischemic ST segment changes [15]. A recombinant fatty acid binding protein bound to a fluorescent tag (ADIFAB) [16;17] has been developed and a second generation assay using a fluorescent molecular probe (ADIFAB2] and a portable reader makes this a potential early marker for the point of care setting. Whilst this marker shows promise in the early phase of ischemia induced ACS, further trials are required to evaluate the diagnosis and prognostic value of FFAu in the chest pain population.

http://dx.doi.org/10.5772/55250

8. Ischemia modified albumin

The NH_2-terminal of human serum albumin (HSA, 66.5 kDa, 585 amino acids) is known to be a binding site for transition metal ions such as cobalt, copper and nickel [18]. Using one and two dimensional 1H-NMR studies, Sadler and colleagues demonstrated binding of Ni^{++}, Cu^{++}, Co^{++}, Cd^{++} and Al^{+++} to bovine and human serum albumin. Strong binding was associated with three N-terminal amino acid residues (Asp-Thr-His in bovine albumin and Asp-Ala-His in human albumin). A Lysine residue designated Lys4 is also involved in the binding site. The authors demonstrated for the fist time selective reduction in the intensities of resonances to the εCH_2 resonance of Lys4 on the addition of Co^{++} to HSA. There are in fact, four metal-binding sites with different specificities in HSA. In addition to the NH_2-terminal, three other sites occur at (i) reduced cysteine at residue Cys34, (ii) site A, including histidine at His67 as a ligand and (iii) the non-localized site B. Cu^{++} and Ni^{++} preferentially bind the NH_2-terminus site. Cd^{++} bind sites A and B, Zn^{++} binds site A and Au^{+} and Pt^{++} bind at residue Cys34.

A reduction in oxygen supply causes localized acidosis and the generation of free radicals. Copper and zinc ions, normally bound to proteins in the plasma are released from protein binding sites to circulate in the free form [19-21]. The N-terminus of albumin binds transition metals. The N-terminus however, is susceptible to biochemical alteration [22]. The altered form is referred to as ischemia modified albumin (IMA). Following a period of ischemia, a reduction in the ability of albumin to bind cobalt is apparent. This is the basis of the albumin cobalt-binding test (ACB® test) for IMA. IMA has been extensively studied in the basic science and clinical research settings and is an FDA cleared CE marked clinical assay for the detection of cardiac ischemia.

It is currently not known if there are any significant changes in total human serum albumin between ischemic and non ischemic patients in the general chest pain population. Many divalent metals bind HSA in the circulation but in concentrations far lower than that required to impact albumin directly. The N-terminal portion of HSA is susceptible to biochemical degradation and is less stable than the albumin of other species [22] including bovine, dog, goat, horse, pig rabbit, rat and sheep but not chicken. Using electrospray-mass spectrometry and N-terminal sequencing, Chan and colleagues have demonstrated degradation corresponding to the first two resides (Asp-Ala) which is dependent both on temperature and the N-terminal alpha-amino group.

IMA however is a form of HSA where the N-terminal amino acids are unable to bind transition metal ions. Myocardial ischemia is known to generate free radicals [21;23], induce localised acidosis [20] and the release of free iron and copper ions bound to enzymes and proteins. [19;24]. Direct evidence of Cu/Fe mobilization in the coronary flow following prolonged (25-60 minute) ischemia but not short (15-21 minute) ischemia has been demonstrated [24]. Both copper and iron concentrations in the first coronary flow fraction were 50-fold and 15-fold higher respectively following prolonged ischemia, compared to pre-ischemic concentrations. This suggests that both copper and iron play a causative role in ischemic cardiac injury by their ability to catalyse the production of free radicals and could be the target of therapeutic intervention to salvage tissue damage [19]. It was therefore postulated that following a period of cardiac ischemia, these processes would result in a change in the ability of the N-terminus of HSA to bind transition metal ions. The release of these ions likely initiates one potential pathway for IMA generation, rather than be considered an interference that may negatively affect IMA. In support of this suggestion, decreased albumin cobalt binding was reported in 99 acute chest pain patients with myocardial ischemia [25] compared to 44 chest pain patients with no evidence of myocardial ischemia. Albumin cobalt binding was also assessed in 41 patients undergoing elective coronary artery angioplasty. Samples were tested using the Albumin Cobalt Binding (ACB) assay before, immediately after, 6 and 24 hours post procedure and compared to results from 13 patients undergoing cardiac catheterization without balloon angioplasty, thus serving as the control group. ACB concentrations were significantly elevated immediately post procedure, compared to the control population and ACB concentrations returned to baseline after six hours [26]; suggesting that HSA undergoes a significant reduction in the capacity to bind exogenous Co^{++} immediately after coronary artery occlusion induced during elective angioplasty. Modification of the Asp-Ala-His-Lys site by N-terminal acetylation or deletion of one or more residues abolishes this cobalt binding [27].

The postulated mechanism (figure 2) of IMA generation is that localised ischemia results in acidosis. The localised acidotic environment stimulates the release of Cu^{++} ions from weak binding sites on circulating proteins such as caeruloplasmin. Caeruloplasmin (EC 1.16.3.1, 151kDa) is a ferroxidase enzyme encoded by the *CP* gene located on Chromosome 3. The enzyme is synthesised in the liver and carries approximately 70% of the total copper in human plasma (a further 15% carried by HSA and the remainder by macroglobulins). Each enzyme molecule contains 6 atoms of copper within its structure.

In the presence of a reducing agent such as ascorbic acid, free copper II is converted to copper I which can react with oxygen to form copper II and generate superoxide free radicals ($O_2\ ^{\bullet-}$). Superoxide dismutase (EC 1.15.1.1) converts the superoxide free radical to hydrogen peroxide which is then degraded by catalase. The copper II ions released are immediately scavenged by human serum albumin but they are tightly bound to the N-terminus. Copper bound albumin is then damaged by hydroxyl free radicals ($OH\ ^{\bullet}$), causing removal of the three N terminal amino acids and release of the copper II ion to repeat the process in a chain reaction [28].Marx and Chevion demonstrated by SDS/polyacrylaminde gel electrophoresis the site specific alteration of HSA in the presence of 50 μM Cu^{++} and increasing portions of 0.2 m Mascorbate; where after the addition of 5 portions, bands at 3, 18, 22, 47 and 50 kDa were observed. The authors also demonstrated that degradation does not occur in the absence of Cu^{++} or in the addition of 1 m Methylenediaminetetraacetic acid (EDTA) or citrate chelating agents [28].

This postulated mechanism, although theoretically attractive has not been borne out in practice. In a study of patients with increased IMA, the N-terminal portion of albumin was sequenced in 8 cases [29] by cleavage of the 11 amino acid resides at the NH_2 terminus, by rapid liquid-phase Edman degradation. The N-terminal amino acid sequence showed normal residues for 6 of 7 patient samples with elevated IMA and one non-ischemic sample (table 1). The remaining patient sample with high IMA demonstrated two missing amino acids at the N-terminus. Clinically this patient did not have an ischemic cardiac event.

http://dx.doi.org/10.5772/55250

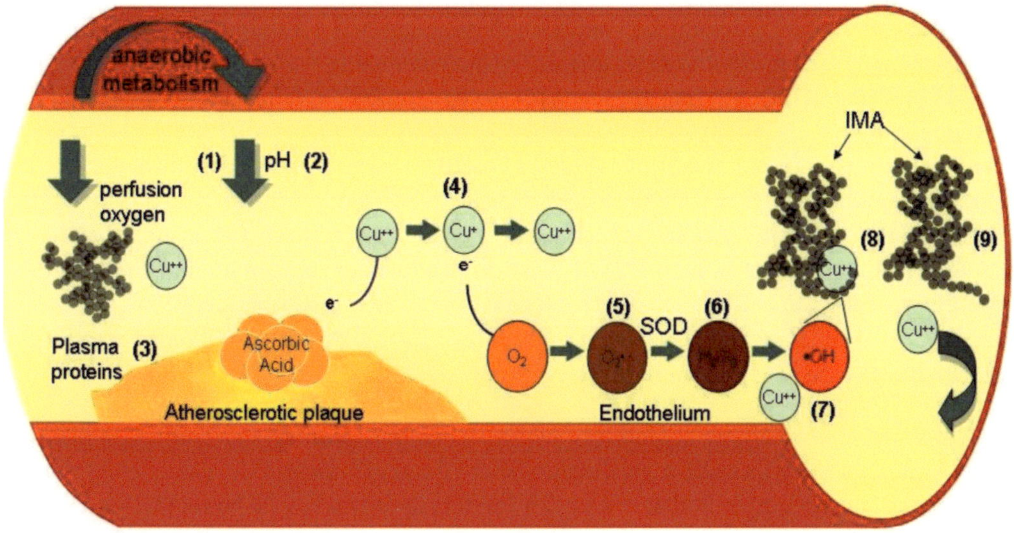

Figure 2. Mechanism of Ischemia Modified Albumin generation. [1]Tissue hypoxia from anaerobic metabolism reduces ATP and causes a [2]lower localized pH inducing acidosis. [3]Cu^{++} ions are released from plasma proteins such as caeruloplasmin. In the presence of ascorbic acid, [4]Cu^{++} is converted to Cu^{+}. Cu^{+} reacts with O_2 to form [5]$O_2^{\bullet -}$. Superoxide dismutase dismutates the $O_2^{\bullet -}$ to [6]H_2O_2, which in presence of Cu^{++} or Fe^{+}, undergoes the Fenton reaction forming [7]OH •hydroxyl radicals. Free Cu^{++} is scavenged by [8]HSA, where it binds tightly to the N-terminus. OH • radicals alter the amino acid N-terminus of [9]HSA rendering it incapable of binding Cu^{++}. These two altered forms are known as IMA.

Subject	NH_2-terminal HSA Sequence
Control (wild type)	DAHKSEVAHRF
Non-ischemic patient, high serum IMA	----HKSEVAHRF
Ischemic patient, high serum IMA	DAHKSEVAHRF
Ischemic patient, high serum IMA	DAHKSEVAHRF
Ischemic patient, high serum IMA	DAHKSEVAHRF
Ischemic patient, high serum IMA	DAHKSEVAHRF
Ischemic patient, high serum IMA	DAHKSEVAHRF
Ischemic patient, high serum IMA	DAHKSEVAHRF

Table 1. Amino (NH_2) terminal sequence analysis of human serum albumin (HAS) from 6 ischemic patients, a control (wild type) and one non ischemic patient with a high serum IMA concentration. (Source: Adapted from Bhagavan et al, ClinChem 2003;49:581-585)

The *in vivo* half-life of HSA is 19-20 days. HSA with a truncated NH_2-terminus would presumably have similar *in vivo* half life properties and yet IMA returns to baseline rapidly after an ischaemic cardiac event. This indicates that the alteration to albumin to create IMA is transient and reversible, rather than a finite chemical alteration. Recent physicochemical studies using electronic absorption EPR and NMR spectroscopy of Co-binding to HSA under anaerobic conditions to prevent Co^{++} oxidation have suggested a different explanation. Using competition experiments with cadmium (Cd^{++}) which binds sites A and B and Cu^{++} which binds the NH_2-terminus, three binding sites for Co^{++} were identified on HSA. Sites A and B showed greater avidity for Co^{++} binding than the NH_2-terminal binding site [30]. Fatty acid binding to albumin occurs at one of the additional cobalt binding sites with a negative allosteric interaction. It is hypothesised, that in myocardial ischemia the release of fatty acids results in binding of fatty acids to albumin. This would then reduce the ability of albumin to take up cobalt hence account for the presence of IMA [30]. If this also produced a conformational change in the albumin affecting the N terminal site, this would also reduce cobalt binding.

8.1. Kinetic release of ischemia modified albumin

Studies in patients receiving angioplasty where ischemia is induced in a controlled manner, have defined the kinetics of IMA production. There is a rapid rise in IMA values after balloon inflation with a subsequent fall at 6 hours and return to normal by 24 hours [31;32]. The rise in IMA occurs earlier than the rise in cardiac troponin and natriuretic peptides (figure 3) and occurs early after the onset of plaque rupture.

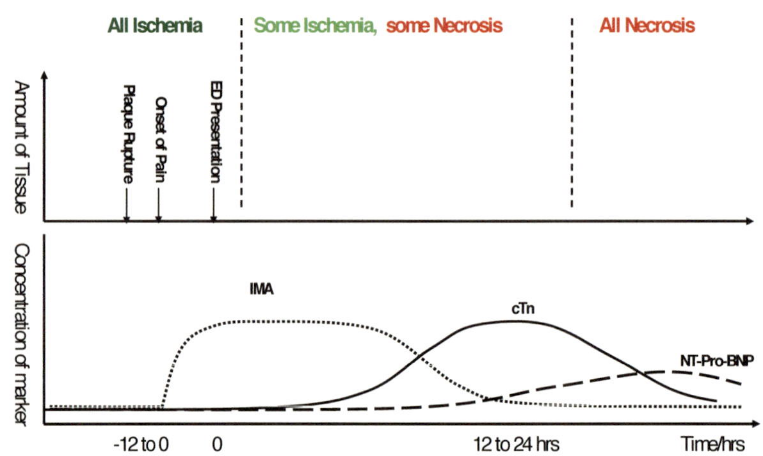

Figure 3. Kinetic release of Ischemia modified albumin (IMA, dotted line) and other cardiac markers, cardiac troponin (cTn, solid line) and natriuretic peptide (NTproBNP, dashed line) [bottom panel], in relation to extent and timing of tissue damage [top panel]

The magnitude of IMA elevation has been found to correlate with the number and frequency of transluminal balloon inflations during the PCI procedure [33]. 34 patients received standard routine care for elective single vessel PCI for the management of stable angina pectoris. 44% of patients received 1-4 balloon inflations whilst, 56% received >5 inflations. IMA concentrations were higher in those with more balloon inflations, higher pressure load of the balloon and the longer the duration of the inflation. IMA is thus not only a marker of the occurrence of ischemia but is also an indicator of the severity of the ischemic episode.

IMA concentrations are lower in patients who demonstrate angiographic evidence of collateral vessels present in the coronary circulation, according to Rentrop's classification [34]. IMA levels post-PCI are higher than baseline, however post-PCI values are lower compared to post-PCI values in those patients without a collateral circulation; irrespective of the extent of coronary artery disease or those who underwent a large number of balloon inflations for longer duration [35]. The lower IMA concentrations in patients with a collateral circulation likely represent a cardioprotective effect against PCI-induced ischemia. IMA elevation is also correlated to the need for subsequent revascularization [36]. Elevated IMA greater than 130 KU/L was associated with a higher frequency of target lesion revascularization at 4-years follow-up in 60 patients who underwent a successful elective single vessel PCI for stable angina pectoris at baseline. The accepted gold standard blood marker for myocardial ischemia is myocardial lactate extraction. Simultaneous IMA and lactate was measured in 10 patients undergoing PCI for chronic stable angina. Post-PCI IMA concentrations paralleled that of transmyocardial lactate [32].

Elevation in serum IMA has been recorded following coronary vasospasm [37]. Twenty six patients with variant angina underwent intracoronary ergonovine spasm provocation testing. Arterial IMA concentrations were measured pre and post procedure and compared to 18 patients undergoing elective PCI and 10 patients with normal coronary angiography. IMA was significantly elevated following drug induced coronary vasospasm compared to baseline and elevated values detected coronary vasospasm with an area under the curve (AUC) of the receiver operating characteristic (ROC) curve of 0.98 (95%CI 0.92-1.00). Other studies involving invasive cardiac procedures have shown rises in IMA where ischemia might occur, occurring concurrently with ECG changes in cardioversion[38], but show a variable picture when there is non-ischemic myocardial damage as in cardiac ablation [39;40].

8.2. Measurement of ischemia modified albumin

The original biochemical test for IMA was known as the albumin cobalt binding (ACB®) assay. This was developed by Ischemia Technologies Inc, Colorado, USA). The assay measures the cobalt binding capacity of albumin in a sample of serum. A known amount of cobalt is added to the patient serum sample. Dithiothreitol (DTT) is added which binds any remaining unbound cobalt and the colorimetric change is measured spectrophotometrically. In serum from non-ischaemic patients, cobalt binds to the N-terminus of HSA, leaving little free cobalt to react with DTT and form a coloured product. Conversely, in serum of patients with ischemia, cobalt does not bind to the N-terminus of modified HSA, leaving more free cobalt to react with DTT and form a darker colour. As normal albumin will bind cobalt, the amount of free cobalt, hence the absorbance will be proportional to the amount of IMA present (figure 4).

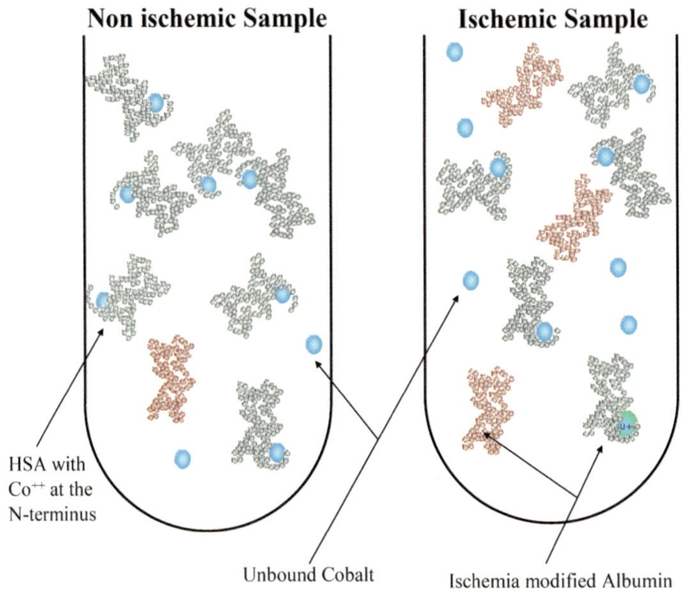

Figure 4. Measurement of Ischemia Modified Albumin by the Albumin Cobalt Binding (ACB) assay. A known amount of $CoCl_2$ is added to a serum sample. DTT is added which binds unbound Co^{++} causing a colorimetric change read spectrophotometrically.

The first generation assay was semi-automated and required a sample pre-treatment step where 500µL of serum sample was added to an Eppendorf tube containing 0.45g $CaCl_2$. The sample was inverted twice and centrifuged at 1200g for 10 minutes. 300µL of supernatant was removed for assay of IMA. For the assay, powdered DTT was provided which required reconstitution in the ratio 15mg DTT: 10 mL diluent. The reconstituted reagent and power required storage at 2-8°C and the working solution had a shelf life of 3-5 days. The second generation of the assay used 7.5mg DTT to 10mL diluent. The third generation assay which became commercially available did not contain the sample pre treatment step and the assay kit contained a concentrated liquid form of DTT which was reconstituted in buffer with a fixed volume 200 µL pipette.

The assay can be performed manually with a spectrophotometer, however it was also initially automated on the Cobas MIRA Plus (Roche Diagnostics) automated spectrophotometer [41]. The assay has since been adapted for other automated clinical chemistry platforms including the LX-20 (Beckman Coulter, Brea, CO, USA) [42], Hitachi 911 (Hitachi, Japan) [43] Hitachi 7600 (Hitachi, Japan) [44] and the Konelab 20 (Thermo Scientific, United Kingdom) [45]. To date a commercialised point of care device for IMA remains to be developed however a pre-commercial portable spectrophotometer and IMA assay has been developed by (Micro-wells Biotechnology Co. Ltd, Shanghai, China). In the Microwells assay, the DTT has been replaced with a stable azo dye chromogen. An automated method to measure ischemia induced alterations of the binding capacity of HSA for nickel [27] has been described [46].

The nickel binding assay correlated well to the ACB assay ($r=0.5387$, $p<0.001$) however the AUC of the ROC curve was higher for the nickel binding assay (0.7582) compared to the ACB assay (0.7289) suggesting nickel binding has a superior ability to discriminate between ACS and non-ACS compared to the ACB assay. There are rumours of an ELISA assay for IMA. This assay is not validated for clinical diagnostic or therapeutic use and an independent performance validation and comparison to the ACB assay does not appear in the current literature. The development of an ELISA however is probably not valid given the rapid alteration and return to baseline of IMA following ischemia, suggesting the alteration is transient and not a permanent change to a specific epitope which could be detected by an antibody.

The *in vitro* stability of the IMA has been shown to be two hours at either 4°C or 20°C, but values increase significantly after four hours irrespective of the storage temperature [33].It is likely that the changes are due to *in vitro* pH changes altering the metal binding capacity of human serum albumin. Samples frozen at -20°C are stable although values have been reported to be slightly higher once thawed, compared to freshly analysed samples [47]. The assay incubation temperature can also affect cobalt binding to HSA and thus influence the IMA concentration [48].

A study of 109 subjects (55 men and 54 women; age range, 20 to 85 years) to determine the 95th percentile reference range for IMA has been performed [49]. The concentrations ranged from 25.7 to 84.5 KU/L with an upper 95th percentile of 80.2 KU/L. This study used the first generation of the assay utilising the pre-handling sample preparation step. Further studies of healthy subjects have reported higher IMA ranges. Abadie and colleagues demonstrated a mean IMA value of 89 KU/L from 69 subjects with a mean age of 49 years [50] whilst Maguire and colleagues demonstrated a 97.5^{th} percentile of 110 KU/L [42] from a population of 81 healthy volunteers (28 men and 53 women aged 22-86 years). Values ranged from 82.0 to 110 KU/L and values were similar between males and females (99.1 vs 100.7 KU/L, $p=0.12$). The biological variation of IMA has been studied [51].In a population of 17 apparently healthy individuals (7 male, 10 female, aged 26-61 years), the within subject coefficient of variation was 2.89% and the between subject coefficient of variation was 6.76%, calculated from weekly blood draws performed at the same time by the same phlebotomist for 5 consecutive weeks. Again there was no specific gender difference in IMA concentrations however the authors reported statistically different IMA concentrations between Caucasian and Black populations, with higher IMA concentrations in Black males and females compared to Caucasian counterparts.

Total serum albumin concentrations might be expected to affect the performance of IMA measurement. There is a relationship between IMA values and serum albumin concentration, although this is much less marked across the reference interval for albumin [52]. The use of an albumin adjusted correction has been proposed [53] although a reference interval study found albumin correction to have little impact compared to other analytical factors [42]. It has been reported that the changes in IMA observed in patients with chest pain was attributable only to changes in the serum albumin concentration [54].

8.3. Clinical utility of ischemia modified albumin in chest pain patients

Clinical validation of any test for ischemia is difficult as there is currently no accepted diagnostic gold standard, although blood lactate has been used previously.In addition, there is no predicate test which can be used against which to perform an initial validation. The initial studies using IMA were based on the ability of an early measurement to predict the final diagnosis of AMI as defined by the elevation of cardiac troponin at 6-12 hours post chest pain. Two studies utilised the first generation pre-release ACB test and a third study manufactured an in-house method. The first study examined acute coronary syndrome (ACS) patients and utilised serial sampling on admission and two subsequent samples [55]. Diagnostic sensitivity of the admission sample for a final diagnosis of AMI was 23.9% for cardiac troponin I (cTnI) alone, 39.1% for IMA alone and 55.9% for the two combined. The second study examined enrolled 256 ACS patients [49]. AUC of the ROC curve for the ACB test was 0.78 with a sensitivity and specificity of 83% and 69% respectively at the optimised decision threshold for AMI. The third study enrolled 75 patients with ischemia and 92 non-ischemic patients [29]. IMA had poor predictive power in discriminating between AMI and non-AMI in patients with underlying ischemic heart disease (AUC of 0.66). However, the test gave good discrimination between patients with or without ischemia. The AUC for the ROC curve for diagnosis of ischemia was 0.95 with sensitivity of 94% and specificity of 88%. In these initial studies there were significant problems with sample stability and the assay involved in addition of calcium chloride and centrifugation as part of the routine method. This made the method unsuitable from routine analysis and the assay was reformulated.

The majority of patients who present to hospital with chest pain and suspected ACS are eventually ruled out for acute myocardial infarction and active unstable coronary disease. The ideal role of an ischemia marker would therefore be as rule out test.The most logical place to use such a test is therefore in the ED.A study of ED presentations examined 208 patients the diagnostic sensitivity of IMA measurement alone was 82% at 46% specificity in samples taken within the first 3 hours. The combination of ECG, cardiac troponin T (cTnT) and IMA showed 95% sensitivity for diagnosis of ACS at presentation [56]. One year follow up performed on this population demonstrated a survival disadvantage in patients with IMA greater than the median concentration of the study group [57]. A subsequent study of 538 patients admitted to a chest pain evaluation unit found admission measurement of IMA plus cTnT had 100% sensitivity for prediction of a final diagnosis of AMI [1]. The presence of an elevated IMA and an elevated cTnT on admission predicted 21% risk of major adverse cardiac events (MACE) compared to patients where both were not elevated, even in patients where the final diagnosis excluded AMI by troponin based criteria. IMA measurement appears to work best as part of a panel of other tests or a test sequence [50]. Admission measurement of IMA has been found to be superior to biomarkers of necrosis and to show 97% sensitivity when combined with them. Not all investigators have considered the diagnostic performance of IMA either alone or in combination with cardiac troponin, or other biomarkers of necrosis, to be adequate. A prospective ED study enrolling 277 patients and using a positive IMA or troponin as the index test and an 8 hour troponin as

http://dx.doi.org/10.5772/55250

the definitive test found only a 97.6% sensitivity with 97% negative predictive value. The investigators did not consider this to be adequate when compared with troponin but did not provide any follow-up data [58]. A second large study prospectively enrolling 189 patients presenting to the ED with chest pain and found an elevated IMA was a poor predictor of cardiac events within the next 72 hours [59]. Conversely, another study found elevated IMA predicted long-term cardiac events [60]. The most consistent finding across all studies of IMA is of a high negative predictive value. This has been highlighted in a meta-analysis specifically examining the role of IMA as a rule out test [61]. The summarised data of over 1800 patients demonstrated a triple negative prediction test (non-diagnostic ECG, negative cTn and negative IMA) with a sensitivity and negative predictive value for ACS of 94.4% and 97.1% respectively.

The prognostic value of IMA in the ACS setting has been investigated [57;60;62;63]. Using a ROC derived cut off of 477 KU/L, Aparci and colleagues found significantly higher mortality at one year in those who had serum IMA >477 KU/L, compared to those with IMA <477 KU/L [60]. Furthermore, using cox regression modelling, IMA was related to mortality, independently of the presence of hypertension, diabetes or advanced age. In a larger cohort of 245 consecutive attendances to the ED, in which there were 31 composite endpoint (cardiac death, AMI or recurrent angina) at 30-days from presentation and 16 deaths at one year; the short and long term ability of IMA to predict outcome was assessed. Short term survival was significantly compromised in those with IMA > 93.3 KU/L compared to those with lower IMA concentrations at both 30 days and 1 year [57]. Using the cohort of the French Nationwide OPERA study IMA, cTn, CRP and BNP were measured within 24hours from admission in 471 patients hospitalized with AMI. Using a primary end point of death, resuscitated cardiac arrest, recurrent AMI or ischemia, heart failure or stroke, 75 in-hospital events and 144 events at 1 year were recorded. Using quartile analysis, 40% of patients reached the end point with IMA concentrations in the highest quartile (>104 KU/L), compared to only 20% of patients in the lowest quartile of 83 KU/L [63]. In those STEMI patients who are treated with primary PCI, IMA is a powerful predictor of 30-day mortality however it does not add to the validated Thrombolysis In Myocardial Infarction (TIMI) risk score [64].

8.4. Clinical utility of ischemia modified albumin in non–chest pain patients

Any marker associated with pathological processes upstream of cardiac necrosis will invariably suffer from a lack of specificity; unlike the cardiac troponins for cardiac necrosis. The further upstream in the ischemic continuum the more likely is the lack of cardiac specificity of the biomarker. Elevations in circulating IMA concentrations are not specific for myocardial ischemia. Mechanistically, IMA can be generated during any ischemic process within the body. A comprehensive review of IMA elevations in non-cardiac conditions is beyond the scope of this chapter but an in-depth summary is given in table 2.Those conditions that have been studied most are explained in more detail below.

Condition
Carbon monoxide poisoning
Congestive cardiac failure
Chronic kidney disease
Deep vein thrombosis
Diabetes Mellitus
Hypercholesterolaemia
Intermittent claudication
Ischemic bowel
Liver cirrhosis
Neural tube defects
Obesity
Pleural effusion
Polycystic ovary syndrome
Polycythemia vera
Preeclampsia
Pulmonary embolism
Skeletal muscle ischemia
Stroke
b-thalassemia
Testicular torsion
Uterine artery embolisation for fibroids

Table 2. Increased serum IMA concentrations in conditions other than acute coronary syndrome.

8.4.1. Skeletal muscle ischemia

Studies of subjects with skeletal muscle ischemia have produced contradictory results. In healthy subjects undergoing arduous physical exertion, IMA has been reported to fall immediately post exercise and then subsequently rise [65-67] or return to normal [68]. Subjects undergoing a forearm ischemia test when the forearm muscles are exercised for 1 minute with the external compression of the arm blood supply showed a fall in IMA, maximal at 3 minutes from the test, returning to baseline by 30 minutes [69]. A similar rise in serum lactate occurred. Conversely during standardized exercise in a plantar flexion pedal combined with inflation of a femoral blood pressure cuff (at 0, 60, 90, 120 and 150 mmHg) to induce calf muscle ischemia an increase in IMA was observed after release of the cuff and returned to baseline within 30 minutes [70]. Peri-operative skeletal muscle ischemia induced by femoral blood pressure cuff being inflated to 300 mmHg in 23 patients undergoing arthroscopic knee surgery. Increased

IMA and myoglobin and decreased albumin were observed following release of the cuff [71]. In patients with peripheral vascular disease (PVD) undergoing a treadmill walk test, a decrease in serum IMA immediately post-test has been documented [72;73]. In 40 consecutive patients undergoing exercise electrocardiography, a significant decrease in IMA at peak exercise then a subsequent rise in IMA has been observed, however there was no difference in IMA concentrations between those patients with positive and negative stress test results [74]. Revascularisation for PVD is accompanied by a post procedural rise in IMA [72;73;75]. In skeletal muscle ischemia, an initial fall with subsequent rise appears to be a consistent finding without adequate explanation. Smooth muscle ischemia does not appear to be associated with a rise in IMA [76]. The effect of skeletal muscle on ischemia will limit the application of IMA measurement after cardiac stress testing for detection of myocardial ischemia and may explain the inconsistent findings[54;74;77;78].

8.4.2. Ischemic stroke

Patients with acute ischemic stroke demonstrate abnormalities in a number of biomarkers of nitrosative and oxidative stress. In 41 patients with ischemic stroke, Senes and colleagues demonstrate that nitrate, IMA and thiobarbituric acid-reactive substances (TBARS) concentrations are significantly increased compared to 37 age and gender matched controls [79]. In a larger cohort of 118 patients presenting within 3 hours of neurological deficit, IMA was elevated in those with cerebral infarction and intracranial haemorrhage (ICH) but normal reference values were observed in those with transient ischemic attacks (TIA) lasting less than 1 hour or those with epileptic seizures [80]. Within 24 hours of injury IMA increased during cerebral infarction but not in intracranial haemorrhage and may offer diagnostic utility in the differential diagnosis of neurological deficit. IMA also correlated with National Institutes of Health Stroke Scale (NIHSS) Score in both cerebral infarction and ICH. Conversely, Herisson and colleagues did not demonstrate a causal relationship between IMA or heart type fatty acid binding protein and NIHSS score or stroke volume [81]. Ahn and colleagues have utilised an albumin-adjusted IMA index for the early detection of ischemic stroke [82]. In 52 patients, 28 (54%) with Ischemic stroke, 24 (46%) non-stroke, the AUC of ROC curve analysis was 0.928 for IMA but 0.99 for albumin-adjusted IMA index. The sensitivity and specificity of the IMA index was superior to IMA concentration alone.

8.4.3. Pulmonary embolus

Pulmonary embolus (PE) is an acute medical emergency estimated to occur in 3.5/1000 hospitalized patients. Patients experience sudden onset dyspnoea, tachypnoea, pleuritic-type chest pain, cyanosis and haemoptysis. PE has an associated mortality of 26%. Diagnosis is primarily based on typical clinical presentation using the Wells and Geneva clinical probability scores. D-dimer measurement and pulmonary angiography are often clinically useful. The ECG can demonstrate acute *corpulmonale* in large PE's but lacks specificity. IMA has been measured in a number of studies of PE patients. Turedi and colleagues [83] have demonstrated that IMA was significantly elevated in 30 PE patients compared to 30 healthy controls and adequately discriminated between the presence and absence of PE. The positive predictive value of IMA for PE is higher than that for D-dimer (79.4% compared to 69.4%) and in combination with the Wells and Geneva criteria, IMA offers an alternative to D-dimer testing [84].

8.4.4. Chronic kidney disease

Patients with chronic kidney disease (CKD) have a reduced life span compared to those without renal disease. Mortality rates are highest in those receiving haemodialysis as renal replacement therapy (RRT). Cardiovascular mortality accounts for the majority of renal deaths. Between 2001 and 2006, 24% of deaths in UK RRT patients were due to ischemic heart disease [85]. This rate is consistent with data from other countries. Cardiovascular morbidity is also increased. 55% of patients receiving haemodialysis RRT also have concomitant congestive cardiac failure. [86]. IMA levels have been determined in patients with CKD [87-89] and in patients receiving haemodialysis (HD) [90-94].

In 2006, Sharma and colleagues demonstrated that patients with elevated IMA have a significantly large left ventricle, decreased systolic function and greater estimated left ventricular filling pressure [88]. Further, in multivariate analysis, a positive dobutamine stress echocardiogram (DSE) combined with elevated IMA and cTnT and E/Ea ratio were independent prognostic factors for death. IMA values increase significantly in those patients with a positive DSE compared to those with no ischemic response [87]. In a modestly small study of 17 anaemic CKD patients and 19 controls, Cichota and colleagues demonstrated that IMA increased in patients compared to the control group. IMA correlated to lactate, haemoglobin and creatinine [89].

Pre and post-HD IMA concentrations are significantly correlated [90], however in this study IMA concentrations were not significantly different between those CKD patients with or without ischemic heart disease, diabetes mellitus or peripheral vascular disease. Fast intravenous iron administration during HD is associated with oxidative stress and inflammation. In a study of 20 HD patients receiving slow intravenous iron administration, IMA concentrations were significantly increased across three HD sessions independently of slow i.v. iron administration [91].Following adjustment of albumin by two methods, post dialysis IMA levels remain significantly increased following HD [92]. Paroxonase-1 (PON-1) is a calcium dependent esterase (arylesterase, aromatic esterase 1, serum aryldialkylpohosphatase 1, EC 3.1.8.1) is a major anti-atherosclerotic component of HDL cholesterol. PON-1 concentrations are lower in CKD patients with and without haemodialysis RRT compared to controls suggesting chronic oxidative stress and accelerated atherosclerosis are a feature of CKD. In a pilot study of CKD patients receiving HD, PON-1 concentrations were significantly and inversely correlated to IMA suggesting an oxidative stress and ischemic process occurs during HD [93]. Recently Albarello and colleagues have evaluated the effect of IMA and protein carbonyl groups as markers of protein oxidation in 23 CKD patients receiving HD. The authors confirm previous reports of higher IMA post-HD than pre-HD and observed a significant correlation between IMA and protein carbonyl groups, attributed to oxidative stress associated with HD [94].

8.4.5. Hyperlipidaemia and obesity

IMA measurement may be of benefit in hypercholesterolaemic patients. IMA is correlated to cholesterol, low density lipoprotein (LDL) and antibodies to oxidised LDL (ox-LDL) [24]. In a study of 37 subjects with hypercholesterolaemia compared to 37 controls, Duarte and colleagues [95] confirm these findings observing IMA correlations to cholesterol, LDL ox-LDL antibodies and to high sensitivity C-reactive protein, suggesting that hypercholesterolaemia is associated with inflammatory and oxidative stress processes, contributing to the advancement of atherosclerosis. IMA is related to the presence of metabolic syndrome independently of age, gender, presence of diabetes or hypercholesterolaemia[96]. Furthermore, the use of 10 mg/day ezetimibe immunotherapy for a duration of 12 weeks in 31 hypercholesterolaemic patients reduced both LDL cholesterol and IMA [97]. The reduction of IMA was independent of the reduction in LDL suggesting that ezetimibe may reduce the burden of oxidative stress in hypercholesterolaemia.

IMA concentrations are higher in obese subjects, with a positive correlation between IMA and body mass index (BMI).In a large study of 148 volunteers in Brazil; subjects were classified as normal, overweight or obese, defined as BMI of 18.5-24.9, 25.0-29.9 and >30 kg/m^2 respectively. IMA concentrations increased exponentially between the three groups, the highest being in those subjects with BMI >30 kg/m^2. Similar findings have been demonstrated in obese post-menopausal women where IMA and IMA: Albumin ratio are higher in those subjects with BMI 26-32 kg/m^2 compared to those with BMI 21-25 kg/m^2. The obese concentrations were similar to those with documented coronary artery disease but normal BMI. In the obese women IMA was positively correlated to BMI, hs-CRP, insulin concentrations and homeostasis assessment model score [98].

8.4.6. Diabetes mellitus

Patients with type 2 diabetes mellitus who demonstrate poor glycaemic control have higher IMA concentrations than those with good glycaemic control. IMA was significantly higher in 76 diabetic patients compared to 25 control subjects and IMA concentrations are correlated to HbA1c [99], glucose and hs-CRP [100]. Conversely, Dahiya and colleagues suggest no significant changes in IMA occur in 60 newly diagnosed type 2 diabetics, compared to 30 control subjects [101]. Diabetic patients who undertake chronic exercise for three months demonstrate lower post exercise IMA concentrations suggesting that exercise alleviates some of the oxidative stress associated with diabetes mellitus [102].

8.4.7. Bowel ischemia

Bowel (mesenteric) ischemia occurs infrequently however if not recognised early, carries a devastatingly high mortality. The presentation is often characterised by generalised abdominal pain, fever, diarrhoea or constipation, tachycardia, hematochezia (blood per rectum), nausea and vomiting. Diagnosis is difficult due to non specific signs and symptoms, plain x-ray or laboratory tests (increased white blood cell count and serum lactic acid). Mesenteric angiography is considered to be the gold standard test which can differentiate between embolic, thrombotic or nonocclusive ischemia. In a preliminary study of 26 patients presenting with symptoms of internal ischemia, Polk and colleagues [103] identified 12 with a positive clinical diagnosis. Positive patients had higher IMA concentrations than those without intestinal ischemia. IMA detected bowel ischemia with a sensitivity of 100% and a specificity of 86%. In a case-controlled study from Turkey, Gunduz and colleagues [104] demonstrated that pre-operative IMA concentrations were significantly higher in patients with thromboembolic occlusion of the superior mesenteric artery (SMA) compared to an age-matched control group of healthy volunteers. A number of animal studies of mesenteric ischemia have provided conflicting results. In a Wistar rat model [105] a time dependent response in IMA in mesenteric ischemia has been demonstrated. 36 mature female rats underwent either simple laparotomy in the control groups or laparotomy followed by clamping of the SMA in the subject group. IMA concentrations were highest 6 hours from ischemic onset, however IMA at 30 minutes and 2 hours were also significantly higher in the clamped group compared to the control group. Elevations of IMA tracked changes in both lactate and malondialdehyde. A similar time dependent change in IMA was demonstrated in New Zealand rabbits undergoing ligation of the SMA compared to either a control group or those undergoing a sham procedure [106]with elevation of IMA at 2 and 6 hours significantly higher than baseline and higher than IMA concentrations in the control rabbits. IMA concentrations mimicked elevations in serum IL-6 with elevated IL-6 in the ischemia group at 1, 3 and 6 hours, but no elevations in the sham operated or control group. In a further study of mesenteric ischemia in a Wistar rat model, Uygun and colleagues [107] demonstrated similar IMA concentrations in control, sham, 2-hour and 6-hour post-SMA ischemia refuting the previous animal studies. It seems likely that IMA may offer additional diagnostic value in the early presentation of mesenteric ischemia. Further prospective studies are required to assess both the diagnostic and prognostic ability of IMA in conjunction with mesenteric angiography to detect bowel ischemia.

8.4.8. Obstetric and gynaecological use of IMA

The care of women and their unborn child during pregnancy is greatly challenging for obstetricians. The adult can interact and provide a history of signs and symptoms whereas the unborn child can only be examined indirectly by means of imaging, foetal heart monitors and a limited number of direct interventions. Women achieving spontaneous preterm (<37 weeks) labour account for 10% of all births and are attributable to 75% of neonatal deaths. The foetus relies entirely on the maternal placenta for O_2/CO_2 exchange. This delicate dependence, between the placenta and the foetus is crucial to normal healthy growth. Any malfunction or disruption to the adequate supply of oxygen can cause hypoxia and potentially fatal acidosis. A limited degree of acidosis is well tolerated by the foetus; however chronic acidosis or hypoxia may lead to a significant mortality and morbidity with potential log-term sequelae. Currently the mechanism of foetal hypoxia and acidosis is unclear, and physiological consequence of foetal acidosis is believed to target the cell energy availability and /or cell poisoning.

During pregnancy plasma proteins change markedly due to increased plasma volume, increased renal blood flow and altered protein synthesis in response to hormonal changes. Plasma volume expansion of up to 45% [1300mL) compared to the non-pregnant state causes an overall net decrease in plasma protein concentration by 10-12 g/L which is reached around week 28 of gestation. The predominant cause of lowered albumin is dilutional, oestrogen is known to affect albumin. The alteration to plasma albumin concentrations throughout the pregnancy period is shown in table 3. The lower concentration of albumin also results in an apparent decrease in substances normally bound to this protein.

Time point	Mean albumin concentration (g/L)	Reference interval (g/L)
Non pregnant control	41	36-46
12 weeks	38	33-43
18 weeks	35	30-39
24 weeks	33	29-37
28 weeks	32	28-37
32 weeks	32	38-36
36 weeks	32	38-36
Full term	32	26-38
1 day post partum	29	23-38
6 weeks post partum	42	37-47

Table 3. Alteration to plasma HSA concentrations during the gestational period.

The HSA reference interval in the full term healthy neonate between term and day 4 is 28-44 g/L. Albumin concentrations increase a little from birth to puberty where the adolescent reference interval (day 4 to 14 years) is 38-54 g/L.

Current experimental studies suggest that foetal development occurs in a hypoxic intrauterine environment and the presence of reperfusion and oxidative stress is believed to be crucial for trophoblast development [108]. Trophoblast invasion of the maternal spiral arteries allows the increase of uterine blood supply necessary to maintain the pregnant state. Serum IMA during normal pregnancy is elevated compared to non-pregnant controls [109-112]. Prefumo and colleagues [109] demonstrate supra-physiological IMA concentrations in early normal pregnancy (11-13 weeks of gestation) suggesting that trophoblast development occurs in a hypoxic uterus. In a large population of 117 pregnant women compared to non-pregnant healthy women, Guven and colleagues demonstrated a cross-sectional elevation in IMA in pregnant women. IMA increased significantly through each trimester. Further, there the authors demonstrated a significant negative correlation between IMA and HSA, suggesting that elevated IMA in pregnancy represents a physiologic state of oxidative stress.

Increased intrauterine hypoxia predisposes to defective endovascular trophoblast invasion of the maternal spiral arteries which may possibly lead to the development of pre-eclampsia; a hypertensive state (>140/90 mmHg) associated with significant proteinuria (≥300mg/dL). Preeclampsia affects 6-8% of pregnancies worldwide. Papageorghiou and colleagues have demonstrated that first trimester serum IMA are significantly higher in women who develop pre-eclampsia compared to those with a normal pregnancy [113]. Both IMA and normalised IMA (IMA: Albumin ratio) were higher in 20 pre-eclamptic women compared to 22 normal pregnancies [112]. These data suggest IMA could be a biological marker of pre-eclampsia however larger studies are required to fully characterise the supra-normal IMA and normalised IMA reference interval in normal pregnancy.

Maternal IMA and normalised IMA concentrations are also increased in women with recurrent pregnancy loss (two or more unexplained miscarriages in the first trimester) compared to healthy pregnancy [114], suggesting that an increase of intrauterine oxidative stress and hypoxia contribute to placental deficiency and subsequently recurrent early miscarriage.

The use of umbilical cord blood for IMA has also been examined. Neonatal cord blood IMA concentrations are higher than IMA concentrations in healthy adults [115] but is not attributable to changes in HSA concentration. Elevated fetal IMA may reflect transient localised ischemia from external forces exerted on the foetus during labour. In a case-control study of 26 newborns, 12 delivered at normal term and 14 with complicated labour or delivered preterm; cord blood IMA concentrations were significantly higher (50%) than those with uneventful deliveries, suggesting IMA is a marker of fetal distress. Doubly-clamped cord blood IMA concentrations are similar in intrauterine growth restriction, compared to those delivered with appropriate for gestational age full-term pregnancies [116]. The similar IMA concentrations may be due to the 'brain sparing effect' accompanied by oligohydraminos (deficiency in amniotic fluid), which is characterised by rerouting the blood supply and the nutrient to vital organs such as the heart, brain and adrenal glands. IMA concentrations in cord blood are higher following caesarean section compared to vaginal delivery and in multigravida compared to primigravida [116] and may be attributable to higher oxidative stress on both accounts. Cigarette smoking during the gestational period alters the oxidant/antioxidant balance in favour of oxidative stress. In response, IMA and MDA concentrations in pregnant smokers are significantly higher and vitamins A and E, SOD and total antioxidant capacityare significantly lower, compared to non-smoking pregnant women [117].

9. Cardiac troponin: Ischemia or necrosis?

The release of cTn was previously thought to occur only in the presence of cell necrosis. The recent development of high sensitivity cTn (hs-cTn) assays has lead to a) the ability to define a true 99th percentile and near-Gaussian distribution in the healthy population and b) earlier diagnosis of AMI with increased sensitivity but at the cost of specificity [118]. A number of clinical and physiological situations have arisen which suggests cTn is released during ischemia in the absence of overt necrosis [119]. These include patients who present with superventricular tachycardia [120] without electrocardiographic changes; in patients with pulmonary embolism [121] where cTn release may indicate a reversible release and under physiological strain following endurance exercise [122]. In all cases the kinetic release is

http://dx.doi.org/10.5772/55250

shortlived with post even values returning to baseline normally within a 24 hour window. Although the mechanisms have not been elucidated postulates include, physiological cardiomyocyte turnover, cellular release of proteolytic degradation products, alteration in plasma membrane permeability and the formation of membranous secretion vesicles containing intracellular derived cTn.

10. Conclusions

Although there are a number of candidate biomarkers for the detection of cardiac ischemia in the research and development world; biomarkers upstream of cardiac cell necrosis lack specificity. They are therefore, at best additive to the diagnostic and prognostic utility of cTn in the early investigation of patients presenting with ischemic type symptoms. The clinical utility of novel biomarkers of ischemia lies in their negative predictive value rather than their ability to adequately rule-in ACS. Given the development of sensitive cTn methods, further work is needed to characterise the release mechanisms of cTn from cardiomyocytes.

Author details

David C. Gaze

Dept of Chemical Pathology Clinical Blood Sciences,St George's Healthcare NHS Trust, London, UK

References

[1] Collinson PO, Gaze DC, Bainbridge K et al. Utility of admission cardiac troponin and "Ischemia Modified Albumin" measurements for rapid evaluation and rule out of suspected acute myocardial infarction in the emergency department. *Emerg Med J*. 2006;23:256-261.

[2] Collinson PO, Gaze DC. Ischaemia-modified albumin: clinical utility and pitfalls in measurement. *J ClinPathol*. 2008;61:1025-1028.

[3] Pope JH, Aufderheide TP, Ruthazer R et al. Missed diagnoses of acute cardiac ischemia in the emergency department. *N Engl J Med*. 2000;342:1163-1170.

[4] Collinson PO, Premachandram S, Hashemi K. Prospective audit of incidence of prognostically important myocardial damage in patients discharged from emergency department. *BMJ*. 2000;320:1702-1705.

[5] Pozen MW, D'Agostino RB, Selker HP et al. A predictive instrument to improve coronary-care-unit admission practices in acute ischemic heart disease. A prospective multicenter clinical trial. *N Engl J Med*. 1984;310:1273-1278.

[6] de Dombal FT, Clamp SE, Softley A et al. Prediction of individual patient prognosis: value of computer-aided systems. *Med Decis Making*. 1986;6:18-22.

[7] Goldman L, Cook EF, Brand DA et al. A computer protocol to predict myocardial infarction in emergency department patients with chest pain. *N Engl J Med*. 1988;318:797-803.

[8] Willems JL, Willems RJ, Bijnens I et al. Value of electrocardiographic scoring systems for the assessment of thrombolytic therapy in acute myocardial infarction. The European Cooperative Study Group for Recombinant Tissue Type Plasminogen Activator. *Eur Heart J*. 1991;12:378-388.

[9] Mathy-Hartert M, Bourgeois E, Grulke S et al. Purification of myeloperoxidase from equine polymorphonuclear leucocytes. *Can J Vet Res*. 1998;62:127-132.

[10] Blair-Johnson M, Fiedler T, Fenna R. Human myeloperoxidase: structure of a cyanide complex and its interaction with bromide and thiocyanate substrates at 1.9 A resolution. *Biochemistry*. 2001;40:13990-13997.

[11] Zhang R, Brennan ML, Fu X et al. Association between myeloperoxidase levels and risk of coronary artery disease. *JAMA*. 2001;286:2136-2142.

[12] Brennan ML, Penn MS, Van Lente F et al. Prognostic value of myeloperoxidase in patients with chest pain. *N Engl J Med*. 2003;349:1595-1604.

[13] Danne O, Mockel M, Lueders C et al. Prognostic implications of elevated whole blood choline levels in acute coronary syndromes. *Am J Cardiol*. 2003;91:1060-1067.

[14] Richieri GV, Kleinfeld AM. Unbound free fatty acid levels in human serum. *J Lipid Res*. 1995;36:229-240.

[15] Kleinfeld AM, Prothro D, Brown DL et al. Increases in serum unbound free fatty acid levels following coronary angioplasty. *Am J Cardiol*. 1996;78:1350-1354.

[16] Richieri GV, Ogata RT, Kleinfeld AM. The measurement of free fatty acid concentration with the fluorescent probe ADIFAB: a practical guide for the use of the ADIFAB probe. *Mol Cell Biochem*. 1999;192:87-94.

[17] Richieri GV, Ogata RT, Kleinfeld AM. A fluorescently labeled intestinal fatty acid binding protein. Interactions with fatty acids and its use in monitoring free fatty acids. *J Biol Chem*. 1992;267:23495-23501.

[18] Sadler PJ, Tucker A, Viles JH. Involvement of a lysine residue in the N-terminal Ni2+ and Cu2+ binding site of serum albumins. Comparison with Co2+, Cd2+ and Al3+. *Eur J Biochem*. 1994;220:193-200.

[19] Chevion M, Jiang Y, Har-El R et al. Copper and iron are mobilized following myocardial ischemia: possible predictive criteria for tissue injury. *Proc Natl Acad Sci U S A.* 1993;90:1102-1106.

[20] Cobbe SM, Poole-Wilson PA. The time of onset and severity of acidosis in myocardial ischaemia. *J Mol Cell Cardiol.* 1980;12:745-760.

[21] McCord JM. Oxygen-derived free radicals in postischemic tissue injury. *N Engl J Med.* 1985;312:159-163.

[22] Chan B, Dodsworth N, Woodrow J et al. Site-specific N-terminal auto-degradation of human serum albumin. *Eur J Biochem.* 1995;227:524-528.

[23] Levine RL. Ischemia: from acidosis to oxidation. *FASEB J.* 1993;7:1242-1246.

[24] Berenshtein E, Mayer B, Goldberg C et al. Patterns of mobilization of copper and iron following myocardial ischemia: possible predictive criteria for tissue injury. *J Mol Cell Cardiol.* 1997;29:3025-3034.

[25] Bar-Or D, Thomas GW, Bar-Or R et al. Diagnostic potential of phosphorylated cardiac troponin I as a sensitive, cardiac-specific marker for early acute coronary syndrome: Preliminary report. *ClinChimActa.* 2005.

[26] Bar-Or D, Winkler JV, Vanbenthuysen K et al. Reduced albumin-cobalt binding with transient myocardial ischemia after elective percutaneous transluminal coronary angioplasty: a preliminary comparison to creatine kinase-MB, myoglobin, and troponin I. *Am Heart J.* 2001;141:985-991.

[27] Bar-Or D, Curtis G, Rao N et al. Characterization of the Co(2+) and Ni(2+) binding amino-acid residues of the N-terminus of human albumin. An insight into the mechanism of a new assay for myocardial ischemia. *Eur J Biochem.* 2001;268:42-47.

[28] Marx G, Chevion M. Site-specific modification of albumin by free radicals. Reaction with copper(II) and ascorbate. *Biochem J.* 1986;236:397-400.

[29] Bhagavan NV, Lai EM, Rios PA et al. Evaluation of human serum albumin cobalt binding assay for the assessment of myocardial ischemia and myocardial infarction. *Clin Chem.* 2003;49:581-585.

[30] Mothes E, Faller P. Evidence that the principal CoII-binding site in human serum albumin is not at the N-terminus: implication on the albumin cobalt binding test for detecting myocardial ischemia. *Biochemistry.* 2007;46:2267-2274.

[31] Collinson PO, Stubbs PJ, Kessler AC. Multicentre evaluation of the diagnostic value of cardiac troponin T, CK-MB mass, and myoglobin for assessing patients with suspected acute coronary syndromes in routine clinical practice. *Heart.* 2003;89:280-286.

[32] Sinha MK, Vazquez JM, Calvino R et al. Effects of balloon occlusion during percutaneous coronary intervention on circulating Ischemia Modified Albumin and transmyocardial lactate extraction. *Heart.* 2006;92:1852-1853.

[33] Quiles J, Roy D, Gaze D et al. Relation of ischemia-modified albumin (IMA) levels following elective angioplasty for stable angina pectoris to duration of balloon-induced myocardial ischemia. *Am J Cardiol*. 2003;92:322-324.

[34] Rentrop KP, Cohen M, Blanke H et al. Changes in collateral channel filling immediately after controlled coronary artery occlusion by an angioplasty balloon in human subjects. *J Am CollCardiol*. 1985;5:587-592.

[35] Garrido IP, Roy D, Calvino R et al. Comparison of ischemia-modified albumin levels in patients undergoing percutaneous coronary intervention for unstable angina pectoris with versus without coronary collaterals. *Am J Cardiol*. 2004;93:88-90.

[36] Dusek J, St'asek J, Tichy M et al. Prognostic significance of ischemia modified albumin after percutaneous coronary intervention. *Clin Chim Acta*. 2006;367:77-80.

[37] Cho DK, Choi JO, Kim SH et al. Ischemia-modified albumin is a highly sensitive serum marker of transient myocardial ischemia induced by coronary vasospasm. *Coron Artery Dis*. 2007;18:83-87.

[38] Conroy S, Kamal I, Cooper J. Troponin testing: beware pulmonary embolus. *Emerg Med J*. 2004;21:123-124.

[39] Roy D, Quiles J, Sinha M et al. Effect of radiofrequency catheter ablation on the biochemical marker ischemia modified albumin. *Am J Cardiol*. 2004;94:234-236.

[40] Sbarouni E, Georgiadou P, Panagiotakos D et al. Ischaemia modified albumin in radiofrequency catheter ablation. *Europace*. 2007;9:127-129.

[41] Gidenne S, Ceppa F, Fontan E et al. Analytical performance of the Albumin Cobalt Binding (ACB) test on the Cobas MIRA Plus analyzer. *ClinChem Lab Med*. 2004;42:455-461.

[42] Maguire OC, O'Sullivan J, Ryan J et al. Evaluation of the albumin cobalt binding (ACB) assay for measurement of ischaemia-modified albumin (IMA) on the Beckman Coulter LX-20. *Ann Clin Biochem*. 2006;43:494-499.

[43] Anwaruddin S, Januzzi JL, Jr., Baggish AL et al. Ischemia-modified albumin improves the usefulness of standard cardiac biomarkers for the diagnosis of myocardial ischemia in the emergency department setting. *Am J Clin Pathol*. 2005;123:140-145.

[44] Su JY, Ju SQ, Wang HM. Measurement of ischemia modified albumin by albumin cobalt binding test. *Chin Med J of Commmunications*. 2005;19:211-214.

[45] Lefevre GF. Analytical performance of the ACB test for ischemia in the Konelab 20. *Clin Chem*. 2003;49:A33.

[46] da Silva SH, Pereira RS, Hausen BS et al. Assessment of the nickel-albumin binding assay for diagnosis of acute coronary syndrome. *Clin Chem Lab Med*. 2011;49:541-546.

[47] Beetham R, Monk C, Keating L et al. Effects of storage at -20 degrees C on ischaemia-modified albumin results. *Ann Clin Biochem*. 2006;43:500-502.

[48] Hausen BS, Signor C, Kober H et al. Effect of temperature on albumin cobalt binding and its influence on ischemia-modified albumin levels in patients with suspected acute coronary syndrome. *Clin Lab*. 2012;58:169-172.

[49] Christenson RH, Duh SH, Sanhai WR et al. Characteristics of an Albumin Cobalt Binding Test for assessment of acute coronary syndrome patients: a multicenter study. *Clin Chem*. 2001;47:464-470.

[50] Abadie JM, Blassingame CL, Bankson DD. Albumin cobalt binding assay to rule out acute coronary syndrome. *Ann Clin Lab Sci*. 2005;35:66-72.

[51] Govender R, De Greef J, Delport R et al. Biological variation of ischaemia-modified albumin in healthy subjects. *Cardiovasc J Afr*. 2008;19:141-144.

[52] Gaze DC, Crompton L, Collinson P. Ischemia-modified albumin concentrations should be interpreted with caution in patients with low serum albumin concentrations. *Med PrincPract*. 2006;15:322-324.

[53] Lee YW, Kim HJ, Cho YH et al. Application of albumin-adjusted ischemia modified albumin index as an early screening marker for acute coronary syndrome. *Clin Chim Acta*. 2007;384:24-27.

[54] van der Zee PM, Verberne HJ, van Straalen JP et al. Ischemia-modified albumin measurements in symptom-limited exercise myocardial perfusion scintigraphy reflect serum albumin concentrations but not myocardial ischemia. *Clin Chem*. 2005;51:1744-1746.

[55] Apple FS, Wu AH, Mair J et al. Future biomarkers for detection of ischemia and risk stratification in acute coronary syndrome. *Clin Chem*. 2005;51:810-824.

[56] Sinha MK, Roy D, Gaze DC et al. Role of "Ischemia modified albumin", a new biochemical marker of myocardial ischaemia, in the early diagnosis of acute coronary syndromes. *Emerg Med J*. 2004;21:29-34.

[57] Consuegra-Sanchez L, Bouzas-Mosquera A, Sinha MK et al. Ischemia-modified albumin predicts short-term outcome and 1-year mortality in patients attending the emergency department for acute ischemic chest pain. *Heart Vessels*. 2008;23:174-180.

[58] Keating L, Benger JR, Beetham R et al. The PRIMA study: presentation ischaemia-modified albumin in the emergency department. *Emerg Med J*. 2006;23:764-768.

[59] Worster A, Devereaux PJ, Heels-Ansdell D et al. Capability of ischemia-modified albumin to predict serious cardiac outcomes in the short term among patients with potential acute coronary syndrome. *CMAJ*. 2005;172:1685-1690.

[60] Aparci M, Kardesoglu E, Ozmen N et al. Prognostic significance of ischemia-modified albumin in patients with acute coronary syndrome. *Coron Artery Dis.* 2007;18:367-373.

[61] Peacock F, Morris DL, Anwaruddin S et al. Meta-analysis of ischemia-modified albumin to rule out acute coronary syndromes in the emergency department. *Am Heart J.* 2006;152:253-262.

[62] Bali L, Cuisset T, Giorgi R et al. Prognostic value of ischaemia-modified albumin in patients with non-ST-segment elevation acute coronary syndromes. *Arch Cardiovasc Dis.* 2008;101:645-651.

[63] Van Belle E, Dallongeville J, Vicaut E et al. Ischemia-modified albumin levels predict long-term outcome in patients with acute myocardial infarction. The French Nationwide OPERA study. *Am Heart J.* 2010;159:570-576.

[64] Dominguez-Rodriguez A, Abreu-Gonzalez P, Jimenez-Sosa A et al. Does ischemia-modified albumin add prognostic value to the Thrombolysis In Myocardial Infarction risk score in patients with ST-segment elevation myocardial infarction treated with primary angioplasty? *Biomarkers.* 2009;14:43-48.

[65] Apple FS, Quist HE, Otto AP et al. Release characteristics of cardiac biomarkers and ischemia-modified albumin as measured by the albumin cobalt-binding test after a marathon race. *Clin Chem.* 2002;48:1097-1100.

[66] Lippi G, Brocco G, Salvagno GL et al. High-workload endurance training may increase serum ischemia-modified albumin concentrations. *Clin Chem Lab Med.* 2005;43:741-744.

[67] Lippi G, Salvagno GL, Montagnana M et al. Influence of physical exercise and relationship with biochemical variables of NT-pro-brain natriuretic peptide and ischemia modified albumin. *Clin Chim Acta.* 2006;367:175-180.

[68] Middleton N, Shave R, George K et al. Novel application of flow propagation velocity and ischaemia-modified albumin in analysis of postexercise cardiac function in man. *Exp Physiol.* 2006;91:511-519.

[69] Zapico-Muniz E, Santalo-Bel M, Merce-Muntanola J et al. Ischemia-modified albumin during skeletal muscle ischemia. *Clin Chem.* 2004;50:1063-1065.

[70] Falkensammer J, Stojakovic T, Huber K et al. Serum levels of ischemia-modified albumin in healthy volunteers after exercise-induced calf-muscle ischemia. *Clin Chem Lab Med.* 2007;45:535-540.

[71] Refaai MA, Wright RW, Parvin CA et al. Ischemia-modified albumin increases after skeletal muscle ischemia during arthroscopic knee surgery. *Clin Chim Acta.* 2006;366:264-268.

[72] Roy D, Quiles J, Sharma R et al. Ischemia-modified albumin concentrations in patients with peripheral vascular disease and exercise-induced skeletal muscle ischemia. *Clin Chem.* 2004;50:1656-1660.

[73] Hacker M, Hoyer HX, la Fougere C et al. Effects of peripheral vascular intervention on ischemia-modified albumin. *Coron Artery Dis.* 2007;18:375-379.

[74] Sbarouni E, Georgiadou P, Theodorakis GN et al. Ischemia-modified albumin in relation to exercise stress testing. *J Am Coll Cardiol.* 2006;48:2482-2484.

[75] Troxler M, Thompson D, Homer-Vanniasinkam S. Ischaemic skeletal muscle increases serum ischaemia modified albumin. *Eur J Vasc Endovasc Surg.* 2006;31:164-169.

[76] Banu NS, Gaze DC, Bruce H et al. Markers of muscle ischemia, necrosis, and inflammation following uterine artery embolization in the treatment of symptomatic uterine fibroids. *Am J Obstet Gynecol.* 2007;196:213-215.

[77] Kalay N, Cetinkaya Y, Basar E et al. Use of ischemia-modified albumin in diagnosis of coronary artery disease. *Coron Artery Dis.* 2007;18:633-637.

[78] Kurz K, Voelker R, Zdunek D et al. Effect of stress-induced reversible ischemia on serum concentrations of ischemia-modified albumin, natriuretic peptides and placental growth factor. *Clin Res Cardiol.* 2007;96:152-159.

[79] Senes M, Kazan N, Coskun O et al. Oxidative and nitrosative stress in acute ischaemic stroke. *Ann ClinBiochem.* 2007;44:43-47.

[80] Abboud H, Labreuche J, Meseguer E et al. Ischemia-modified albumin in acute stroke. *Cerebrovasc Dis.* 2007;23:216-220.

[81] Herisson F, Delaroche O, Auffray-Calvier E et al. Ischemia-modified Albumin and Heart Fatty Acid-binding Protein: Could Early Ischemic Cardiac Biomarkers Be Used in Acute Stroke Management? *J Stroke Cerebrovasc Dis.* 2010.

[82] Ahn JH, Choi SC, Lee WG et al. The usefulness of albumin-adjusted ischemia-modified albumin index as early detecting marker for ischemic stroke. *Neurol Sci.* 2011;32:133-138.

[83] Turedi S, Gunduz A, Mentese A et al. Value of ischemia-modified albumin in the diagnosis of pulmonary embolism. *Am J Emerg Med.* 2007;25:770-773.

[84] Turedi S, Gunduz A, Mentese A et al. The value of ischemia-modified albumin compared with d-dimer in the diagnosis of pulmonary embolism. *Respir Res.* 2008;9:49.

[85] The Renal Association. UK Renal Registry Report. 2007.

[86] National Institutes of Health NIoDaDaKD. US Renal Data System, USRDS 2007 Annual Data Report: Atlas of Chronic Kidney Disease and End-Stage Renal Disease in the United States. 2007.

[87] Sharma R, Gaze DC, Pellerin D et al. Evaluation of ischaemia-modified albumin as a marker of myocardial ischaemia in end-stage renal disease. *Clin Sci (Lond).* 2007;113:25-32.

[88] Sharma R, Gaze DC, Pellerin D et al. Ischemia-modified albumin predicts mortality in ESRD. *Am J KidneyDis.* 2006;47:493-502.

[89] Cichota LC, Moresco RN, Duarte MM et al. Evaluation of ischemia-modified albumin in anemia associated to chronic kidney disease. *J Clin Lab Anal.* 2008;22:1-5.

[90] Montagnana M, Lippi G, Tessitore N et al. Effect of hemodialysis on traditional and innovative cardiac markers. *J Clin Lab Anal.* 2008;22:59-65.

[91] Malindretos P, Sarafidis PA, Rudenco I et al. Slow intravenous iron administration does not aggravate oxidative stress and inflammatory biomarkers during hemodialysis: a comparative study between iron sucrose and iron dextran. *Am J Nephrol.* 2007;27:572-579.

[92] Kiyici A, Mehmetoglu I, Karaoglan H et al. Ischemia-modified albumin levels in patients with end-stage renal disease patients on hemodialysis: does albumin analysis method affect albumin-adjusted ischemia-modified albumin levels? *J Clin Lab Anal.* 2010;24:273-277.

[93] Kotani K, Kimura S, Gugliucci A. Paraoxonase-1 and ischemia-modified albumin in patients with end-stage renal disease. *J Physiol Biochem.* 2011;67:437-441.

[94] Albarello K, Dos Santos GA, Bochi GV et al. Ischemia modified albumin and carbonyl protein as potential biomarkers of protein oxidation in hemodialysis. *Clin Biochem.* 2012.

[95] Duarte MM, Rocha JB, Moresco RN et al. Association between ischemia-modified albumin, lipids and inflammation biomarkers in patients with hypercholesterolemia. *Clin Biochem.* 2009.

[96] Valle Gottlieb MG, Da Cruz IB, Duarte MM et al. Associations among metabolic syndrome, ischemia, inflammatory, oxidatives, and lipids biomarkers. *J Clin Endocrinol Metab.* 2010;95:586-591.

[97] Kotani K, Caccavello R, Sakane N et al. Influence of ezetimibemonotherapy on ischemia-modified albumin levels in hypercholesterolemic patients. *Pharmacol Rep.* 2011;63:1248-1251.

[98] Kazanis K, Dalamaga M, Kassi E et al. Serum levels of ischemia modified albumin in overweight/obese postmenopausal women: a potential biomarker of atherosclerotic burden associated with oxidative stress. *Maturitas.* 2011;70:182-187.

[99] Piwowar A, Knapik-Kordecka M, Warwas M. Ischemia-modified albumin level in type 2 diabetes mellitus - Preliminary report. *Dis Markers.* 2008;24:311-317.

[100] Kaefer M, Piva SJ, De Carvalho JA et al. Association between ischemia modified albumin, inflammation and hyperglycemia in type 2 diabetes mellitus. *Clin Biochem*. 2010;43:450-454.

[101] Dahiya K, Aggarwal K, Seth S et al. Type 2 diabetes mellitus without vascular complications and ischemia modified albumin. *Clin Lab*. 2010;56:187-190.

[102] Kurban S, Mehmetoglu I, Yerlikaya HF et al. Effect of chronic regular exercise on serum ischemia-modified albumin levels and oxidative stress in type 2 diabetes mellitus. *Endocr Res*. 2011;36:116-123.

[103] Polk JD, Rael LT, Craun ML et al. Clinical utility of the cobalt-albumin binding assay in the diagnosis of intestinal ischemia. *J Trauma*. 2008;64:42-45.

[104] Gunduz A, Turedi S, Mentese A et al. Ischemia-modified albumin in the diagnosis of acute mesenteric ischemia: a preliminary study. *Am J Emerg Med*. 2008;26:202-205.

[105] Gunduz A, Turkmen S, Turedi S et al. Time-dependent variations in ischemia-modified albumin levels in mesenteric ischemia. *Acad Emerg Med*. 2009;16:539-543.

[106] Dundar ZD, Cander B, Gul M et al. Serum ischemia-modified albumin levels in an experimental acute mesenteric ischemia model. *Acad Emerg Med*. 2010;17:1233-1238.

[107] Uygun M, Yilmaz S, Pekdemir M et al. The diagnostic value of ischemia-modified albumin in a rat model of acute mesenteric ischemia. *Acad Emerg Med*. 2011;18:355-359.

[108] Jauniaux E, Hempstock J, Greenwold N et al. Trophoblastic oxidative stress in relation to temporal and regional differences in maternal placental blood flow in normal and abnormal early pregnancies. *Am J Pathol*. 2003;162:115-125.

[109] Prefumo F, Gaze DC, Papageorghiou AT et al. First trimester maternal serum ischaemia-modified albumin: a marker of hypoxia-ischaemia-driven early trophoblast development. *Hum Reprod*. 2007;22:2029-2032.

[110] van Rijn BB, Franx A, Sikkema JM et al. Ischemia modified albumin in normal pregnancy and preeclampsia. *Hypertens Pregnancy*. 2008;27:159-167.

[111] Guven S, Alver A, Mentese A et al. The novel ischemia marker 'ischemia-modified albumin' is increased in normal pregnancies. *Acta Obstet Gynecol Scand*. 2009;88:479-482.

[112] Gafsou B, Lefevre G, Hennache B et al. Maternal serum ischemia-modified albumin: a biomarker to distinguish between normal pregnancy and preeclampsia? *Hypertens Pregnancy*. 2010;29:101-111.

[113] Papageorghiou AT, Prefumo F, Leslie K et al. Defective endovascular trophoblast invasion in the first trimester is associated with increased maternal serum ischemia-modified albumin. *Hum Reprod*. 2008;23:803-806.

[114] Ozdemir S, Kiyici A, Balci O et al. Assessment of ischemia-modified albumin level in patients with recurrent pregnancy loss during the first trimester. *Eur J ObstetGynecol-Reprod Biol.* 2011;155:209-212.

[115] Gugliucci A, Hermo R, Monroy C et al. Ischemia-modified albumin levels in cord blood: a case-control study in uncomplicated and complicated deliveries. *Clin Chim Acta.* 2005;362:155-160.

[116] Iacovidou N, Briana DD, Boutsikou M et al. Cord blood ischemia-modified albumin levels in normal and intrauterine growth restricted pregnancies. *Mediators Inflamm.* 2008;2008:523081.

[117] SongulSahinli A., Marakoglu K, Kiyici A. Evaluation of the levels of oxidative stress factors and ischemia modified albumin in the cord blood of smoker and non-smoker pregnant women. *J Matern Fetal Neonatal Med.* 2011.

[118] Gaze DC. High-sensitive cardiac troponin assays: application for prime-time use. *Biomark Med.* 2010;4:341-343.

[119] White HD. Pathobiology of troponin elevations: do elevations occur with myocardial ischemia as well as necrosis? *J Am Coll Cardiol.* 2011;57:2406-2408.

[120] Redfearn DP, Ratib K, Marshall HJ et al. Supraventricular tachycardia promotes release of troponin I in patients with normal coronary arteries. *Int J Cardiol.* 2005;102:521-522.

[121] Muller-Bardorff M, Weidtmann B, Giannitsis E et al. Release kinetics of cardiac troponin T in survivors of confirmed severe pulmonary embolism. *Clin Chem.* 2002;48:673-675.

[122] Shave R, BaggishA, George K et al. Exercise-induced cardiac troponin elevation: evidence, mechanisms, and implications. *J Am Coll Cardiol.* 2010;56:169-176.

Chapter 7

Is Hyperuricemia a Risk Factor to Cardiovascular Disease?

Magda H M Youssef

Additional information is available at the end of the chapter

http://dx.doi.org/10.5772/54871

1. Introduction

Uric acid is a weak acid distributed throughout the extracellular fluid compartments (Emmerson, 1996). The normal blood uric acid level in humans is approximately 4 mg/dl (0.24 mmol/l) (Ganong, 2005). Uric acid is the end product of purine degradation. Purines are degraded ultimately to uric acid through the action of the enzyme xanthine oxidase that converts xanthine to urate (Mc Lean, 2003). In most mammals, the liver enzyme uricase (urate oxidase) is responsible for further metabolism of uric acid to allantoin, which is more soluble waste product. However, humans lack the enzyme uricase, resulting in higher blood uric acid levels (Hediger et al., 2005). They might provide humans a survival advantage over the other primates because of the function of uric acid as antioxidant (Mc Lean, 2003).). For an individual, urate concentration is determined by the balance between the rate of purine metaboloism, both endogenous and exogenous, and the efficiency of renal clearance. Alteration in this balance may account for hyperuricemia. In the majority (90%) of patients with primary gout, hyperuricemia results from relative renal undersecretion, whereas in 10% of patients, there is overproduction of endogenous uric acid (Fam, 2002).

Elevated serum uric acid, besides its documented link to gouty arthritis, has been reported to be closely-associated with the metabolic syndrome and, as well, to be a correlate of the development and progression of cardiovascular diseases (Baker et al., 2005), though the role of uric acid in this respect is still unclear. Several possible pathological mechanisms linking hyperuricemia to cardiovascular disease were suggested; including the deleterious effects of elevated uric acid on endothelial dysfunction, oxidative metabolism, as well as platelet adhesiveness, hemorheology and aggregation (Hoieggen et al., 2003). However, no enough or definite experimental data exist concerning the association of hyperuricemia with the different cellular elements of blood. The aim of this work was to investigate the effects of elevated serum uric acid levels on the physiology of the different cellular blood elements in rats and their link to cardiovascular ailment.

2. Methods

This study was performed on 58 albino rats, of both sexes, weighing 180- 250g. Rats included in the present study were divided into 2 main groups: hyperuricemic group (group I) and normouricemic control group (group II). Hyperuricemia was achieved by using the uricase inhibitor oxonic acid (oxonic acid, potassium salt, supplied by Acros Organics, Geel, Belgium), with concomitant supplementation of diet with 3% uric acid. Oxonic acid was administered orally for 5 days, 2 and 4 weeks by gavage in a dose of 750 mg/kg body weight (Khosla et al., 2005), dissolved in 0.25% methylcellulose. Concomitant supplementation of diet with uric acid was done to obtain better and maintained hyperuricemic response (Mazzali et al., 2001). The control groups were received the solvent orally for 5 days, 2 and 4 weeks. Studied rats were allocated into the following groups and subgroups: Group I: Hyperuricemic rats, that received the oxonic/uric acid regimen. Rats in this group were further subdivided into 3 subgroups according to the duration of hyperuricemia: Group Ia: Five-days hyperuricemic rats (n=10), receiving the oxonic/uric acid regimen for 5 consecutive days. Group Ib: Two-weeks hyperuricemic rats (n=11), receiving the regimen 6 days/week for 2 weeks. Group Ic: Four-weeks hyperuricemic rats (n=10), receiving the regimen 6 days /week for 4 weeks. Group II: Normouricemic control rats, that received methylcellulose, the solvent for oxonic acid, orally by gavage. Rats in this group were further subdivided into 3 subgroups, matching the hyperuricemic subgroups:

Group IIa: Five-days control rats (n=8), receiving the solvent for five consecutive days. Group IIb: Two-weeks control rats (n=8), receiving the solvent 6 days/week for 2 weeks. Group IIc: Four-weeks control rats (n=11), receiving the solvent 6 days/week for 4 weeks.

Experimental procedure: At the end of the experimental period, overnight fasted rats were weighed and anaesthetized with intraperitoneal injection of sodium thiopental (40 mg/kg body weight). One ml of blood was drawn into a tube containing EDTA for assessment of complete blood picture. Three ml of blood was collected in a chilled plastic tube containing sodium citrate 3.8%, gently mixed for assessment of platelet aggregation. Another blood samples were collected in chilled plastic tubes containing sodium citrate 3.8gm/100 ml (9 volumes of blood to 1 volume of sodium citrate) and gently shaken. These blood samples were used for study of platelet aggregation. The citrated blood was centrifuged at 1500 r.p.m. for 5 min. The supernatant platelet rich plasma (PRP) was pipetted into clean plastic tubes. The remaining blood sample was centrifuged at 10,000 r.p.m. for 10 min. to prepare platelet poor plasma (PPP). Standard PRP: the number of platelets in PRP was counted using coulter T-660 counter. The platelet number was adjusted to a standardized number of 3×10^5 platelet per μl by dilution with autologus platelet poor plasma.

Aggregation study: platelet aggregation was performed using Chrono-Log automatic aggregometer (model 540-VC, Chrono-Log Corp, Harvertown, USA) coupled with computer and printer. ADP as an aggregating agent was used at a final concentration of 10 uM. The maximum aggregation was recorded after 3 min. Platelet aggregation was tested by the turbidimetric technique, according to the method of Mustard et al. (1964). Platelet aggregation was induced in stirred platelet-rich plasma (PRP) by addition of the aggregating agent ADP (Park com). The platelet count in PRP was adjusted to a standardized number of 3x105 platelet/μl by dilution with autologus platelet poor plasma to obtain standard PRP. Platelet aggregation was performed by the use of a chrono-Log automatic aggregometer (model 540, chrono-Log Corporation, Harvertown, USA), coupled with computer and printer.

Enzymatic determination of plasma uric acid was carried out according to the method of Barhan and Trinder (1972). Nitrate concentration in plasma was estimated according to the method described by Bories and Bories (1995). C-reactive protein (CRP) was determined qualitatively by the use of latex slide test, described by Singer et al. (1957).

3. Results

Administration of oxonic/uric acid regimen for 5 days, 2 and 4 weeks resulted in a highly significant hyperuricemic response, being less marked in the 4-weeks treated group. This observation could be explained by increased urinary uric acid excretion in the later group. Hediger et al. (2005) demonstrated increased mRNA transcription of the urate transporters ($URAT_1$) in association with hyperuricemia. No significant changes were found as regard erythrocyte parameters, platelet count or mean platelet volume between hyperuricemic and control groups.

As regards the leucocyte changes accompanying hyperuricemia, the neutrophil% was significantly increased and lymphocyte % was significantly decreased compared to control values despite the non-significant changes in the total leucocytic count. Neutrophils were speculated to liberate a potent activation signal after interaction with monosodium urate crystals, and that this activation can further stimulate surrounding neutrophils and contribute to amplification of the inflammatory response, with the redox pathways being implicated in these reactions (Desaulniers et al., 2006). Further, C-reactive protein, the systemic inflammatory marker, was markedly increased in the 2- and 4-weeks hyperuricemic rats compared to controls. Uric acid was reported to induce expression of CRP in vascular endothelial and smooth muscle cells, which was proposed to provide a pathogenic link to explain the association of the systemic inflammatory response and elevated uric acid in patients with cardiovascular disease and diabetes.(Kang et al., 2005; Saito et al., 2003). The increased neutrophil %, and the significant positive correlation observed between uric acid level and neutrophil %, together with the increased CRP, encountered in the present study, support the previous findings of Ruggiero et al.(2006) pointing to significant and independent association of uric acid level with neutrophil count and CRP level. On the other hand, the lymphocyte % was significantly reduced in all the hyperuricemic groups. The encountered lymphocytopenia could be attributed to the increased free radical burden in hyperuricemia, leading to increased lymphocyte apoptosis. Uric acid has been demonstrated to act in some instances as prooxidant, generating free radicals (Patterson et al., 2003).

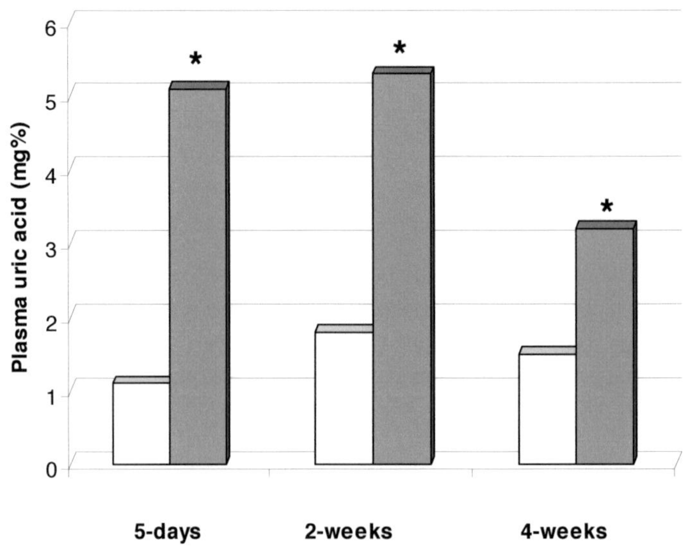

Figure 1. changes in plasma uric acid in the different hyperuricemic groups [grey box] and their matching control groups [white box]

With regard to platelet changes associated with hyperuricemia, enhanced ADP-induced platelet aggregation was encountered in all the hyperuricemic groups compared to controls, the effect being more marked in the 5-days and 2-weeks groups, showing higher uric acid levels. Moreover, a significant positive correlation between plasma uric acid and platelet aggregation was demonstrated in all the tested groups of rats. The observed enhancement of platelet aggregation is in accordance with previous reports (Alderman and Aiyer, 2004).

The enhanced platelet aggregation demonstrated in the present study could be explained by many mechanisms. Urate crystals were reported to stimulate arachidonic acid metabolism in platelets.(Serhan et al., 1984) Moreover, neutrophilia demonstrated in the present study might contribute to platelet hyperaggregability, as neutrophils were reported to be potent inducers of platelet Ca^{2+} flux, aggregation and secretion. (Faint, 1992). Furthermore, the observed lymphocytopenia could play a role in the increased platelet activity. In 1987, Wu et al. proposed lymphocytes to possess PGI_2 synthase activity which is capable of converting platelet-derived PGH_2 into PGI_2 that is sufficient to inhibit platelet function. Therefore, the encountered decrease in lymphocytes could provide an additional explanation for the enhanced platelet aggregability.

The observed decrease in plasma nitrate level in the 4-weeks hyperuricemic rats, together with the significant negative correlation between plasma levels of uric acid and nitrate demonstrated in this group, reflect possible lowering of nitric oxide (NO) bioavailability with prolongation of hyperuricemia. Reduced NO production in association with hyperuricemia has been reported by several investigators.(Waring and Esmail, 2005) The reduced NO, together with the inflammatory response, could imply increased risk of cardiovascular pathology in hyperuricemic subjects by promoting development of endothelial dysfunction.

In conclusion, the neutrophil and platelet activation, known predisposing factors to thrombosis, together with increased CRP production and reduced NO production, might share in causing the hyperuricemia-associated endothelial dysfunction and atherosclerotic plaque formation. Therefore, it could be recommended that physicians should be aware of the role of elevated uric acid in inducing cardiovascular insult, and that individuals suffering from hyperuricemia should be advised to have a strict follow-up for their platelet function, which could participate in the cardiovascular pathology.

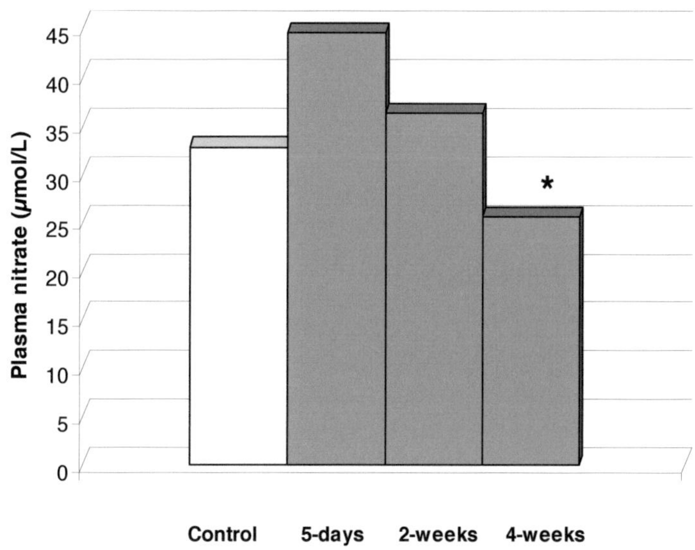

Figure 2. changes in plasma nitrate in the normouricemic ☐ and the different hyperuricemic groups ☐

Duration Parameter	5-days hyperuricemia			2-weeks hyperuricemia			4-weeks hyperuricemia		
	Control rats	Hyper-uricemic rats	P	Control rats	Hyper-uricemic rats	P	Control rats	Hyper-uricemic rats	P
TLC ($x10^3/\mu l$)	3.2±0.38 (7)	3.0±0.56 (9)	NS	2.8±0.39 (7)	3.2±0.59 (9)	NS	3.7±0.52 (9)	3.9±0.76 (10)	NS
Neutrophil (%)	31.6±2.93 (7)	53.1±3.87 (9)	<0.001	34.4±4.25 (7)	56.9±6.92 (9)	<0.05	35.0±7.25 (9)	58±6.42 (10)	<0.05
Lymphocyte %	67.6±3.37 (7)	46.2±4.00 (9)	<0.01	64.3±4.12 (7)	41.0±7.17 (9)	<0.05	64.6±7.23 (9)	41.5±6.33 (10)	<0.05

Table 1. Results of the changes in leucocyte parameters in the different studied groups **P**: Significance of difference from matched control rats calculated by Student's "t"test for unpaired data. **NS**: Not significant.

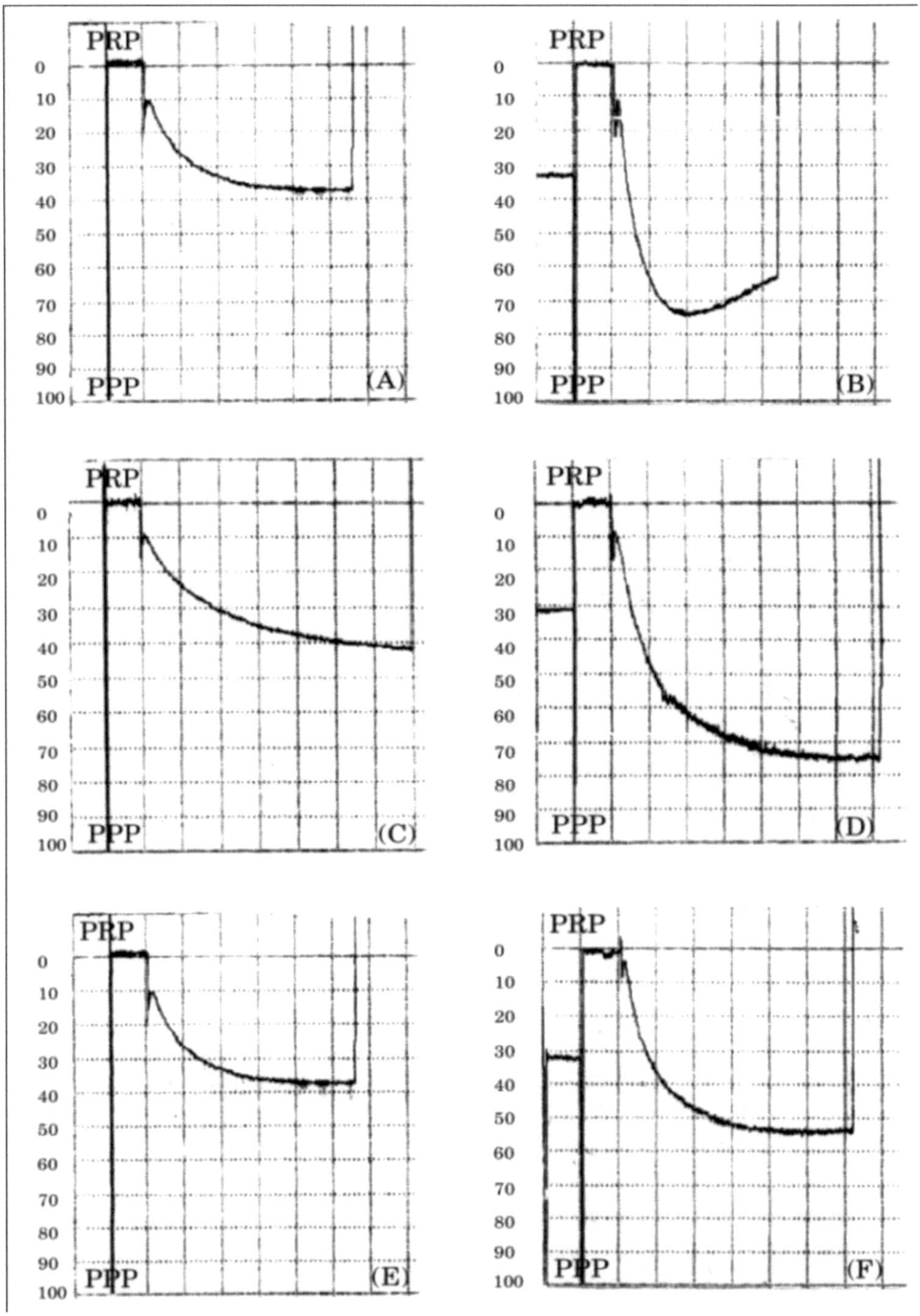

Figure 3. Tracing of ADP-induced platelet aggregation in the different studied groups; 5 days normouricemic rats (A), hyperuricemic rats for 5 days (B), normouricemic rats for 2 weeks (C), hyperuricemic rats for 2 weeks (D), normouricemic rats for 4 weeks (E) and hyperuricemic rats for 4 weeks (F).

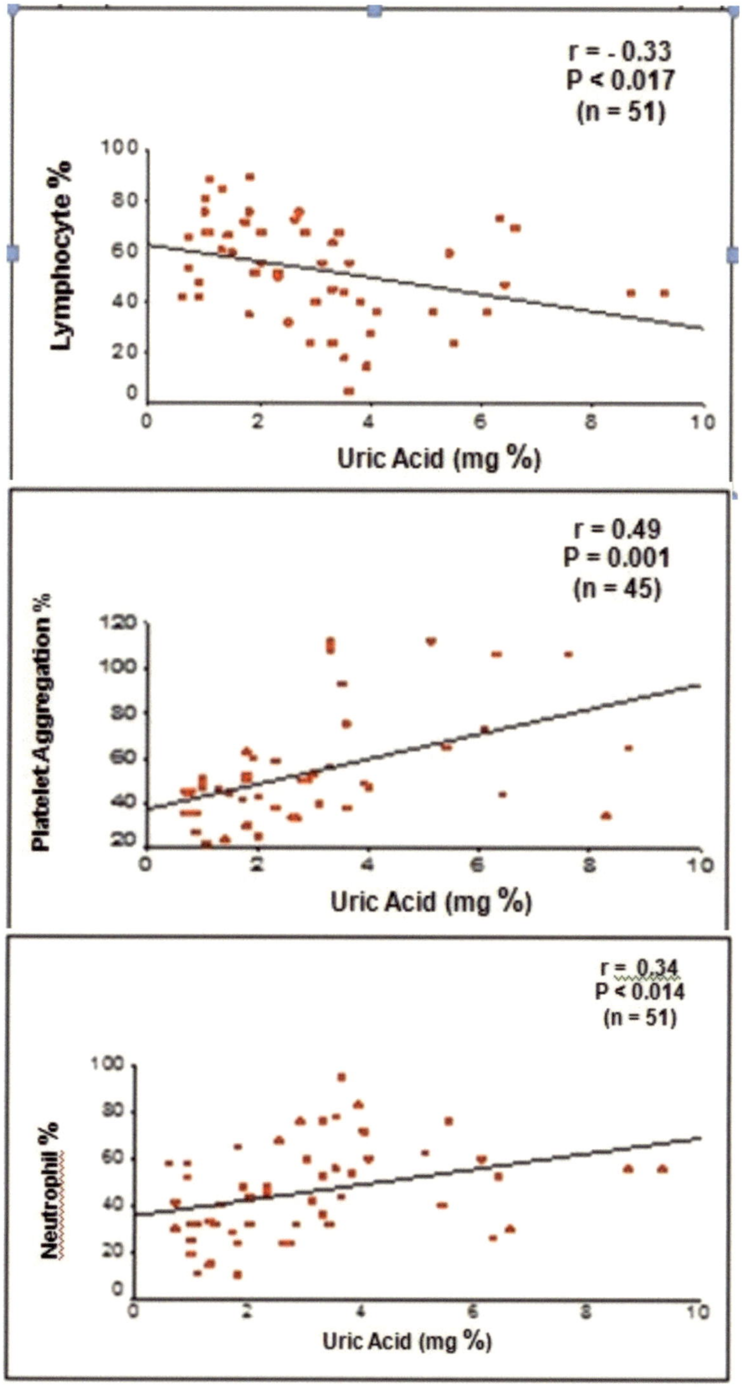

Figure 4. Graphs showing correlations of plasma uric acid versus neutrophil %, lymphocyte%, and platelet aggregation in all the studied groups of rats.

Author details

Magda H M Youssef

Physiology Department, Faculty of Medicine, Ain Shams University, Cairo, Egypt

References

[1] Alderman, M, & Redfern, J. S. (2004). Serum uric acid-a cardiovascular risk factor? Ther Umsch; 61:547.

[2] Baker, J. F, Krishnan, E, Chen, L, & Schumacher, H. R. (2005). Serum uric acid and cardiovascular disease: Recent developments, and where do they leave us? Am J Med; 118:816.

[3] Barhan, D, & Trinder, P. (1972). An improved colour reagent for the determination of blood glucose by the oxidase system. Analyst; 97:142.

[4] Bories, N. P, & Bories, C. (1995). Nitrate determination in biological fluids by an enzymatic one step assay with nitrate reductase. Clin Chem; 41:904.

[5] Desaulniers, P, Marois, S, Popa-nita, O, Gillbert, C, & Naccache, P. H. (2006). Characterization of an activation factor released from human neutrophils after stimulation by triclinic monosodium urate crystals. J Rheumatol;33:928.

[6] Emmerson, B. T. (1996). The management of gout. New England J Med; , 334, 445-51.

[7] Faint, R. W. (1992). Platelet-neutrophil interactions: their significance. Blood Rev; 6:83.

[8] Fam, A. G. (2002). Gout, diet, and the insulin resistance syndrome. J Rheumatol; , 29, 1350-5.

[9] Ganong, W. F. (2005). Energy Balance, Metabolism, and Nutrition. In: Review of Medical Physiology, 22th edition. McGraw-Hill, United State of America., 297-298.

[10] Hediger, M. A, Johnson, R. J, Miyazaki, H, & Endou, H. (2005). Molecular Physiology of urate transport. Physiology; , 20, 125-33.

[11] Hediger, M. A, Johnson, R. J, Miyazaki, H, & Endou, H. (2005). Molecular physiology of urate transport. Physiology; 20:125.

[12] Hoieggen, A, Fossum, E, Reims, H, & Kjeldsen, S. E. (2003). Serum uric acid and hemorheology in borderline hypertensives and in subjects with established hypertension and left ventricular hypertrophy. Blood Press; 12:104.

[13] Kang, D. H, Han, L, Ouyang, X, Kahn, A. M, Kanellis, J, Li, P, Feng, L, Nakagawa, T, Watanabe, S, Hosoyamada, M, Endou, H, Lipkowitz, M, Abramson, R, Mu, W, &

Johnson, R. J. (2005). Uric acid causes vascular smooth muscle cell proliferation by entering cells via a functional urate transporter. Am J Nephrol; 25:425.

[14] Khosla, U. M, Zharikov, S, Finch, J. L, Nakagawa, T, Roncal, C, Mu, W, Krotova, K, Block, E. R, Prabhakar, S, & Johnson, R. J. (2005). Hyperuricemia induces endothelial dysfunction. Kidney Inter; 67:1739.

[15] Mazzali, M, Hughes, J, Kim, Y, Jefferson, J. A, Kang, D, Gordon, K. L, Lan, H. Y, Kivlighn, S, & Johnson, R. J. (2001). Elevated uric acid increases blood pressure in the rat by a novel crystal-independent mechanism. Hypertension; 38:1101.

[16] Mc Lean, L. (2003). The pathogenesis of gout. In: Rheumatology. Hochberg, M.C., Ginsberg, M.H., Kozin, F., O'Malley, M. & McCarty, D.J. (eds.), Mosby, New York., 1903-1918.

[17] Mustard, J. F, & Hegard, T. B. RowSell, H.C. ((1964). Effects of adenosine nucleotides on platelets aggregation and clotting time. J Lab Clin Med; 64:548.

[18] Patterson, R. A, Horsley, E. T, & Leake, D. S. (2003). Prooxidant and antioxidant properties of human serum ultrafiltrates toward LDL: Important role of uric acid. J Lipid Res; 44: 512.

[19] Ruggiero, C, Cherubini, A, Ble, A, Bos, A. J, Maggio, M, Dixit, V. D, Lauretani, F, Bandinelli, S, Senin, U, & Ferrucci, L. (2006). Uric acid and inflammatory markers. Euro Heart J; 27: 1174.

[20] Saito, M, Ishimitsu, T, Minami, J, Ono, H, Ohrui, M, & Matsuoka, H. (2003). Relation of plasma high-sensitivity C-reactive protein to traditional cardiovascular risk factors. Atherosclerosis; 167:73

[21] Serhan, G. C, Lunberg, U, Weissmann, G, & Samuelsson, B. (1984). Formation of leukotriens and hydroxyl acids by human neutrophils and platelets exposed to monosodium urate. Prostaglandins; 4:563.

[22] Singer, J. M, Pratz, C. M, Pader, E, & Elster, S. K. (1957). The latex fixation test: Agglutination test for C-reactive protein and comparison with the capillary precipitin method. Am J Clin Pathol; 28:614.

[23] Waring, W. S, & Esmail, S. (2005). How should serum uric acid concentrations be interpreted in patients with hypertension? Curr Hypertens Rev; 1:89.

[24] Wu, K. K, Papp, A. C, Manner, C. E, & Hall, E. R. (1987). Interaction between lymphocytes and platelets in the synthesis of prostacyclin. J Clin Invest; 6:1601.

Chapter 8

Patient on ACS Pathway – Hypomagnesaemia a Contributory Factor to Myocardial Ischemia

Ghulam Naroo, Tanveer Ahmed Yadgir,
Bina Nasim and Omer Skaf

Additional information is available at the end of the chapter

http://dx.doi.org/10.5772/55286

1. Introduction

Magnesium is the 4th most abundant intracellular cation in the body. Normal adult plasma concentration ranges from 1.7 to 2.5 mg/dL. Most of the body's reserves are found in the skeletal bone mass.

Hypomagnesaemia is a common electrolyte abnormality seen in around 12% hospitalized patients and has an incidence as high as 60 to 65 % in Intensive Care Unit patients.

Clinical signs and symptoms are only possible in severe magnesium deficiency. Surprisingly, magnesium depletion can present despite a near normal serum magnesium level.

Common nutritional sources include green leafy vegetables, legumes, nuts, animal proteins, seafood and sea greens like kelp.

Absorption takes place in the upper small intestine, where nearly 30 to 50% of consumed magnesium is taken up depending upon the endogenous magnesium status.

Magnesium is excreted by the kidneys.

In circulation 33% is albumin bound (non-filterable), 12% complexed with anions & 55% is in the free ionized form (filterable fraction)

2. Magnesium at cellular level

Magnesium serves as a cofactor for over 300 enzymes involved in Deoxyribonucleic Acid (DNA) and Ribonucleic Acid (RNA) synthesis, protein synthesis, energy metabolism and maintenance of electrical potential of nervous tissue and cell membranes.

Of particular importance is the role of this element in regulating potassium fluxes through Sodium (Na) Pottasium (K) ATPase pump and involvement in metabolism of Calcium. (*Magnesium is a natural calcium channel blocker)*

Na K Pump – the sodium potassium pump is activated by magnesium. With magnesium deficiency there is impaired pump activity, whereby insufficient potassium can be pumped into the cell, although the supply may be great enough.

The energy substrate for the transport activity of the sodium/potassium pump is represented by Adenosine Triphosphate (ATP) in form of its magnesium complex. This ATP-Mg^{++} complex is split by the ATPase delivering the transport energy and therefore it is said that the ATPase is directing the sodium/potassium pump.

Furthermore with Magnesium deficiency there is not enough energy substrate. Hence the cell membrane shows increased permeability and the potassium gradient cannot be maintained.

Potassium leaves the cell, in compensation sodium and hydrogen influx takes place passively. Magnesium leaves the cell, if not enough ATP is present for forming the ATP-Mg complex and calcium influx will follow.

Calcium (Ca) Pump and Na/Ca exchange - There are two possibilities for elimination of calcium out of the cell, but unfortunately both are impaired by magnesium deficiency:

They are the calcium pump and the sodium/calcium exchange.

Calcium pump- After muscle contraction calcium ions will be transported back again from the cytosol to the stores of the sarcoplasmatic reticulum by the calcium pump. The concentration gradient at this action needs a high expense of energy: one ATP for two calcium ions. The calcium transport-ATPase is magnesium dependent.

Sodium calcium exchange-. During the action potential calcium influx takes place along the slow calcium channels into the cell and induces the contraction process. The calcium influx will be compensated again by an exchange of three sodium ions into the cell. The energy for the exchange originates from the high extracellular sodium concentration, but these three sodium-ions must be removed again out of the cell by the sodium/potassium pump which requires one ATP. If the performance of the sodium/potassium pump is impaired, cellular sodium will increase and inhibit sodium/calcium exchange. This can be due to ATP deficiency, myocardial ischemia/ reperfusion injury, potassium/ magnesium deficiency.

Increased sodium within the cell results in hypertension and the increased calcium within the cell increases the vascular tone in the smooth muscle of the artery to aggravate the hypertension.

http://dx.doi.org/10.5772/55286

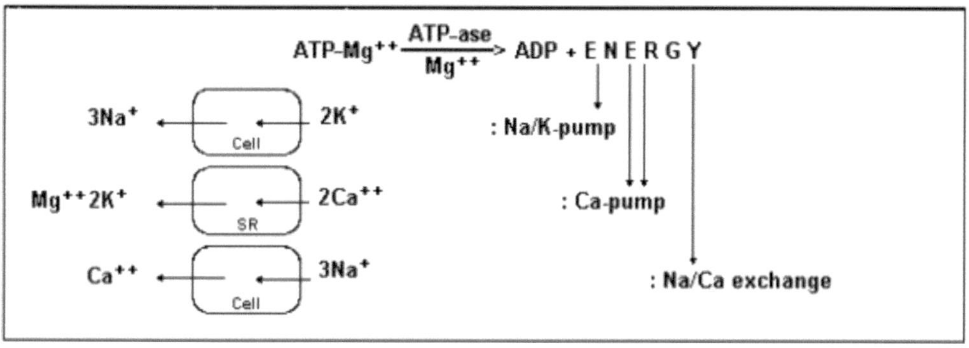

Figure 1. ATP-Mg++ : Energy Supply for pumps and exchange

3. Causes of hypomagnesaemia

Pathologic effects of primary nutritional deficiency of magnesium is rare unless a relatively low magnesium intake is accompanied with prolonged diarrhea or excessive urinary magnesium losses.

Gastrointestinal Causes-

- Acute/ Chronic Diarrhea
- Malabsorption syndromes
- Steatorrhea
- Small bowel bypass
- Inborn errors of metabolism – autosomal recessive disorder, chromosome 9, selective defect in magnesium absorption due to a mutation in gene that encodes for a member of receptor channel family.
- Acute pancreatitis – Saponification of magnesium and potassium ions.

Renal Causes-

- Loop and thiazide diuretics – cause mild hypomagnesaemia, because volume contraction increase proximal sodium, water and magnesium reabsorption
- Alcoholics- Alcohol induced tubular dysfunction which is reversible within 4 weeks.
- Hypercalcemia- increased filtered calcium load competes with magnesium in transport across the ascending limb of loop of Henle.
- Nephrotoxins- Aminoglycosides, amphotericin B, cisplatin, cyclosporine
- Loop of Henle & Distal tubule dysfunction – Barters Syndrome and Gitelmans syndrome.

4. Effects of hypomagnesaemia on tissues

- Hypokalemia- Hypokalemia induced due to deficiency of magnesium is refractory to potassium supplementation until magnesium deficiency is corrected.
- Hypocalcaemia- due to diminished secretion of Parathyroid hormone and resistance to the effect of parathyroid hormone at the receptor level. Parathyroid hormone (PTH) induced release of calcium from bone is impaired when plasma Mg < 0.8 mg/ dL.
- Vitamin D Deficiency- Low plasma level of Calcitriol is noted in Hypomagnesaemia which further contributes to Hypocalcaemia.

5. Clinical manifestations of hypomagnesaemia

- Cardiac Effects - Arrhythmias, Heart Disease
- Metabolic Effects - Hypokalemia, Hypocalcemia, Diabetes, Osteoporosis
- Neurological Effects– Headache, paresthesias, tremors, muscular spasms, tetany, convulsions, migraine, irritability, anxiety, weakness, mood swings, depression.
- ECG Changes-

Initial stage- widening of QRS Complex peaking of T waves

Later stage- prolongation of PR interval, progressive widening of QRS complex and diminution of T wave.

6. Diagnosis of magnesium deficiency

The serum magnesium level correlates poorly with total body stores. As a result, there have been several intracellular assays of magnesium from lymphocytes, red blood cells, and muscle biopsies. These assays include nuclear magnetic resonance (NMR) spectroscopy and ion-specific electrode measures. But since these tests are very expensive, therefore they are not clinically applicable at present. For these reasons, despite its limitations serum magnesium levels are commonly and easily carried out to evaluate the magnesium status. If the serum magnesium level is low, intracellular magnesium is also low but it is important to understand that many patients may have normal serum magnesium levels but may still be intracellularly depleted. [1]

7. Discussion

Low serum magnesium is an independent predictor of CHD in both gender. Although relation exist more in women and less in men. A cross-sectional cohort study has shown inverse association between serum magnesium and carotid intima-media thickness(12.). Low serum magnesium causes endothelial damage that accelerates the atherosclerotic process leading to ACS. Evidence links significant low serum magnesium to CHD in patient with Acute Myocardial Infarction (AMI) versus control [13] [14]. This cohort of 15,792 middle aged subjects were assessed over a four to seven year period as part of the Atherosclerosis Risk in Communities (ARIC) study [2]. The relative risk of CHD across quartiles of serum magnesium was 1.0 (in the lowest quartile), 0.92, 0.48 and 0.44. Both men and women who developed CHD had lower mean baseline serum magnesium concentration than the disease-free controls.

Another study of 50 patients with coronary heart disease found that oral magnesium supplement therapy improved endothelial function and exercise tolerance compared to placebo. Autopsy has shown that magnesium concentrations in cardiac muscle of individuals who died of heart disease is lower than those of accident victims [15] [16] One study, found a 20% reduction in magnesium in the non-infarcted and a 50% reduction in the infarcted myocardium. Also infarcted myocardium had a depressed magnesium/calcium ratio [16]. A prospective National Health and Nutritional Examination Survey (NHANES) I follow up study showed the important role of modifiable dietary and behavioral characteristics in the causation and prevention of coronary heart disease hospitalization and mortality. This study was done over a 10 years follow up of 8251 subjects. The study emphasized the role of modifiable dietary factors including magnesium as well as behavioral characteristics in the causation and prevention of CHD [17].

Another epidemiologic study showed an inverse association between dietary magnesium and incident CHD. These associations were present after adjustment for multiple confounding factors, including race, smoking, alcohol intake, life style & exercise, waist/hip ratio, fibrinogen & lipids level, diuretics use and HRT [17]. Diabetes and hypertension may merely be confounders but low magnesium concentration may contribute to the pathogenesis of diabetes or hypertension [18] [19]· High intake of foods rich in magnesium including green vegetables, nuts and whole grains may provide protection against CHD by increasing magnesium levels [20]

The following effects of magnesium might play an important role in protecting the myocardium in patients of Unstable Angina:

- Reducing the ischemic myocardial death by reducing the intracellular calcium overload by limiting the reperfusion injury.
- Dilating the coronary arteries. [21]
- Reducing the after load. [22]
- Inhibiting the platelet function by its effect on prostacyclin secretion.
- Attenuating the catecholamine release by reducing the sympathetic activity. [23]

Other effects of magnesium beneficial in myocardial infarction and life threatening ventricular arrhythmias include the above and following:

- Direct antiarrhythmic effect.

- Reducing free radical formation.
- Enhanced collateral flow.

Magnesium has been shown to inhibit calcium influx in the cell, it reduces the mitochondrial calcium overload, conserves the intracellular ATP as Mg2+-ATP, and raising extracellular magnesium has been shown to be protective in ischemia. Magnesium inhibits the spasm of the coronary arteries [21], increases the coronary blood flow, and decreases the coronary vascular resistance in patients of Variant Angina. This can be a direct effect of magnesium on coronary vasculature or it can be an indirect effect by reducing the catecholamine release.

High catecholamine levels play an important role in the pathogenesis and prognosis of unstable angina and are closely related to the extension of an infarct [24]. Magnesium tends to inhibit the release of catecholamines from the adrenal medulla and reduces the sensitivity of a- adrenergic receptors to catecholamines, thereby reducing the arrythmogenic and the pressor effects of the catecholamines [25]. Deficiency of magnesium therefore enhances the sympathetic activity and increases the catecholamine induced myocardial damage.

A double blind randomized placebo controlled study was conducted to assess the 24 hour infusion of magnesium in patients of unstable angina [26]. In this study the patients who presented with unstable angina and had electrocardiographic changes were randomized to receive 24hour intravenous infusion of magnesium or placebo within 12hr of admission. The chosen primary endpoints in this study included ECG changes as assessed by 48h Holter monitoring, resting 12 lead ECGs, CK-MB release and urinary catecholamine levels.

In this study patients were followed for 1month. Thirty-one patients received magnesium sulphate and 31 placebo. Baseline characteristics and extent of coronary disease were similar in both groups. On 48 h Holter monitoring, 14 patients(50%) were found to have transient ST segment shifts in the magnesium group versus 12 patients (46%) in the placebo group. However, there were fewer ischemic episodes in the magnesium group (51 versus 101, P<0001) and there was a trend towards an increase in the total duration of ischemia in the placebo group compared to the magnesium group in the second 24 h. It was found that regression of T wave changes on the 24 h ECG and reduction in the ST segment changes in the 12 lead ECG, occurred more frequently in patients who received magnesium compared to those treated with placebo (11 patients versus 0 patients respectively, P<0005).

Creatine kinase-MB release was significantly less at 6 and 24 h in patients who received magnesium compared to those treated with placebo. Catecholamine excretion was lower in patients treated with magnesium than in those treated with placebo in the first 12 h sample, *P<005).* On continuous ECG monitoring, a similar proportion of patients in each treatment group had evidence of myocardial ischemia in the first 24 h of recording. However, the number of episodes was significantly less in the magnesium group and the number of patients with transient myocardial ischemia in this group fell from 11 patients (39%) to five (18%) in the second 24 h of recording with no change in the placebo group (10 patients [39%] in both the first and second 24 h).

This study concluded that magnesium infusion reduces the ischemic ECG changes, cardiac markers, and urinary catecholamine excretion in the acute phase of unstable angina. Therefore magnesium is useful in these patients.

Among the other studies which have suggested that magnesium may reduce mortality and serious arrhythmias post acute myocardial infarction is the Second Leicester intravenous magnesium intervention trial (LIMIT-2) study [27], which was a double-blind randomized trial of 2316 patients with suspected acute MI who received either intravenous magnesium sulfate or placebo along with other currently accepted therapies for MI, including thrombolysis. Thirty-five percent of the patients received a fibrinolytic agent, usually streptokinase, and 66 percent received aspirin. The presence of an acute MI was confirmed in 65 percent of cases.

An important design feature of this trial was that magnesium was administered **prior** to a fibrinolytic agent. A treatment effect was observed in all subgroups, including those receiving thrombolysis and it showed a 24% reduction in mortality, 25% reduction in the incidence of left ventricular failure and 21% reduction in the mortality from ischemic heart disease.

In another small trial which revealed a positive association of magnesium to coronary heart disease, 194 patients with an acute MI who were not considered candidates for fibrinolytic therapy were randomized to receive either intravenous magnesium sulfate or placebo. In this study the benefits of magnesium compared to placebo showed a reduction in the in-hospital mortality especially in the elderly and a lower incidence of both arrhythmias and left ventricular dysfunction.

However, this was not supported by the results of International Study of Infarct Survival (ISIS-4) study [28] which showed that a 24-h infusion of magnesium has no beneficial effect in those receiving thrombolysis for acute myocardial infarction. In this study, patients were randomized after the thrombolytic agent had been administered, a mean of 8 h after the onset of pain, compared to a median of 3 h in the Leicester intravenous magnesium intervention trial (LIMIT-2) trial, in which iv magnesium was given prior to thrombolysis. Animal studies have shown that the effect of magnesium is greatest if given before spontaneous or induced reperfusion, as this reduces the reperfusion induced myocardial injury, and this may account, in part, for the lack of benefit seen in International Study of Infarct Survival (ISIS-4).

8. Conclusion

Data suggest that hypomagnesemia may precede CHD. The U.S. National Academy of Sciences has estimated that a nation-wide initiative to add calcium and magnesium to soft water might reduce the annual cardiovascular death rate by 150,000 in the United States. [7]. It is recommended to design further observational and interventional studies to substantiate the link.

Author details

Ghulam Naroo[1], Tanveer Ahmed Yadgir[2], Bina Nasim[3] and Omer Skaf[4]

1 Emergency & Trauma Centre, Rashid Hospital Dubai, United Arab Emirates

2 Research & Accreditation Department, Dubai Corporation for Ambulance Services, Dubai, United Arab Emirates

3 Rashid Hospital, Dubai, United Arab Emirates

4 Dubai Corporation for Ambulance Services, Dubai, United Arab Emirates

References

[1] Altura, B. M, Brodsky, M. A, Elin, R. J, et al. Magnesium: growing in clinical importance. Patient Care (1994). , 10, 130-150.

[2] Liao, F, Folsom, A. R, & Brancati, F. L. Is low magnesium concentration a risk factor for coronary heart disease? The Atherosclerosis Risk in Communities Study. Am Heart J (1998).

[3] Taneva, E. Hypokaliaemia and hypomagnesemia during acute coronary syndrome: A- 661. European Journal of Anaesthesiology (2005). , 22-issue, 172.

[4] Altura, B. M. Aimin Z Altura BT: Magnesium, hypertensive vascular disease, atherogenesis, subcellular compartmentation of calcium and magnesium and vascular contractility. Miner Electrolyte Metab (1993). , 19, 323-336.

[5] Paolisi, G. Barbagallo M: Hypertension, diabetes, and insulin resistance: the role of intercellular magnesium. Am J Hypertension (1997). , 10, 346-355.

[6] Chester Fox MD, Delano Ramsoomair, MD, and Cathleen Carter, PhD: Magnesium: Its Proven and Potential Clinical Significance. South Med J. (2001).

[7] http:/ / www.mgwater.com/, The Magnesium website.(2002). access dated- 27/11/12)

[8] Oral Mg therapy improves endothelial function in pt with ACSShechter M,Sharir Circulation.(2000).

[9] The important role of modifiable dietary and behavioral characterisics in the causation and prevention of coronary heart disease hospitalization and mortality; the perspective NHANES follow up study, Gartside PS, Glueck CJ Jam Coll Nutr.(1995).

[10] 10. Antman, EM, Anbe, DT, & Armstrong, PW. ,et al. ACC/AHA guidelines for the management of patients with ST-elevation myocardial infarction.

[11] Redwood, S. R, Basir, Y, Huang, J, et al. Effect of magnesium sulphate in patients with unstable angina. A double blind,randomized,placebo-controlled study.Eu Heart J (1997).

[12] Ma, J, Folsom, A. R, Melnick, S. L, Eckfeldt, J. H, Sharrett, A. R, Nabulsi, A. A, et al. Associations of serum and dietary magnesium with cardiovascular disease, hypertension, diabetes, insulin, and carotid arterial wall thickness: the ARIC Study. J Clin Epidemiol (1995). , 48, 927-40.

[13] Singh, R. B, Rastogi, S. S, Ghosh, S, & Niaz, M. A. Dietary and serum magnesium levels in patients with acute myocardial infarction, coronary artery disease and noncardiac diagnoses. J Am Coll Nutr (1994). , 13, 139-43.

[14] Kafka, H, Langevin, L, & Armstrong, P. W. Serum magnesium and potassium in acute myocardial infarction: influence on ventricular arrhythmias. Arch Intern Med (1987). , 147, 465-9.

[15] Marier, J. R. Water hardness, human health and the importance of magnesium. Ottawa: National Research Council of Canada. NRCC Series (1979). (17581), 65-84.

[16] Speich, M, Bousquet, B, & Nicolas, G. Concentrations of magnesium, calcium, potassium, and sodium in human heart muscle after acute myocardial infarction. Clin Chem (1980). , 26, 1662-5.

[17] The role of modifiable dietary and behavioral characteristics in the causation and prevention of coronary heart disease hospitalization and mortality- NHANES follow up study-1.

[18] White JR Jr. Campbell RK. Magnesium and diabetes: a review. Ann Pharmacother (1993). , 27, 775-80.

[19] 31. Resnick, L. M. Cellular calcium and magnesium metabolism in the pathophysiology and treatment of hypertension and related metabolic disorders. Am J Med (1992). A):11S-20S.

[20] 48. Fraser, G. E, Sabate, J, Beeson, W. L, & Strahan, T. M. A possible protective effect of nut consumption on risk of coronary heart disease: the Adventist Health Study. Arch Intern Med (1992). , 152, 1416-24.

[21] Vigorito, C, Giordano, A, Ferraro, P, et al. Hemodynamic effects of magnesium sulfate on the normal human heart. AmJ Cardiol (1991). , 67, 1435-7.

[22] Rasmussen, H, Larsen, O, Meier, K, & Larsen, J. Hemodynamic effects of intravenously administered magnesium on patients with ischemic heart disease. Clin Cardiol (1988). , 824-8.

[23] James, M, Cork, R, Harlen, G, & White, J. Interactions of adrenaline and magnesium on the cardiovascular system of the baboon. Magnesium (1988).

[24] Penny, W. J. The deleterious effects of myocardial catecholamines on cellular electrophysiology and arrhythmias during ischaemia and reperfusion. Eur Heart J (1984). , 5, 960-73.

[25] Bean, B, & Varghese, P. Role of dietary magnesium deficiency in the pressor and arrhythmogenic response to epinephrine in the intact dog. Am Heart J (1994). , 127, 96-102.

[26] Redwood Sr, Bashir Y, Huang J. Effect of magnesium sulfate in patients of unstable angina. European heart journal (1997).

[27] Woods Kl, Flether S. Long term outcome after intravenous magnesium sulfate in suspected acute myocardial infarction. The second Leicester intravenous magnesium intervention trial. LIMIT-2. Lancet (1994).

[28] ISIS-4the Fourth International Study of Infarct Survival- Lancet (1995).

Chapter 9

Cell Autophagy and Myocardial Ischemia/Reperfusion Injury

Suli Zhang, Jin Wang, Yunhui Du, Jianyu Shang, Li Wang, Jie Wang, Ke Wang, Kehua Bai, Tingting Lv, Xiao Li and Huirong Liu

Additional information is available at the end of the chapter

http://dx.doi.org/10.5772/53442

1. Introduction

Ischemic heart disease is a clinical syndrome resulting from myocardial ischemia and is characterized by an imbalance between the supply and demand of myocardial blood flow and myocardial oxygen metabolism. It is currently one of the major diseases that endanger human health. Early and effective reconstruction of ischemic myocardial blood perfusion is the fundamental measure taken to prevent the development of ischemic myocardial injury, reduce myocardial infarct size, and improve the clinical prognosis. However, several studies have discovered that in some cases, reperfusion of ischemic cells could cause further injury in the form of ischemia/reperfusion injury. The clinical manifestations of myocardial ischemia-reperfusion injury include arrhythmia, myocardial stunning, and no-reflow. Although lethal reperfusion injury in clinical practice is more difficult to identify, it is the most serious consequence of ischemia/reperfusion injury and is also the main reason preventing the ischemic myocardium recovery from effective reperfusion therapy. Therefore, studies on the modes of myocardial cell death after ischemia/reperfusion are of great significance. Previous studies suggested that myocardial cell death following myocardial ischemia/reperfusion injury were mainly necrosis and apoptosis. Apoptosis receives more attention due to its death program. However, in recent years, a number of studies have suggested that, another procedural manner of death---autophagy, type II programmed cell death, also plays a critical role in ischemia/reperfusion injury. The study of this death pathway may provide a new effective way to block myocardial ischemia/reperfusion injury. Therefore, in this chapter, the roles and possible mechanisms of autophagy in myocardial ischemia/reperfusion injury will be reviewed.

2. Definition, formation and classification of autophagy

In 1962, Ashford and Porter discovered the 'self-eating' phenomenon in liver cells using an electron microscope [1]. After that, this process was named autophagy by Duve, a Belgian cellular biologist and chemist [2].

Autophagy is the transportation and degradation of damaged, denatured or aged proteins. It is a common cellular physiological process which can maintain cell homeostasis. Autophagy is an evolutionary conserved pathway of self-digestion that occurs in various eukaryotic organisms from yeast to mammals [3]. It is also a cellular defense mechanism in many pathological processes. The autophagy process time is relatively short (T1/2 for 8 mins), it illustrates that autophagy is an effective response to environmental changes for cells, and it plays a pivotal role in metabolism: (1) Since autophagy is an adaptive response to exogenous stimuli (including nutritional deficiencies, the cell density load, hypoxia, oxidative stress, infection, etc.), and its products of degradation, such as amino acids, nucleotides, and free fatty acids, can participate in the material and energy cycle; (2) As a housekeeper mechanism for cells to maintain a steady state, autophagy can adjust the renovation of long-lived proteins, peroxisomes, mitochondria and endoplasmic reticulum; (3) Autophagy is involved in tissue-specific integration; (4) Autophagy can act as a defense mechanism to remove the damaged cytoplasm and metabolites, and the reconstruction on the subcellular level can protect the affected cells. Meanwhile, as a cell death procedure, autophagy can induce cell initiative death [4].

Although autophagy and autophagy-related processes are dynamic, they can be broken down into several discrete steps. There are four steps in autophagy: induction, formation of autophagosomes, formation of autolysosomes and degradation of the content. Autophagy serves as a response to stress such as nutrient limitation, and this is one of its primary roles in unicellular organisms such as yeast. Then, portions of cytoplasm are first isolated (sequestered) within a double membrane enclosed vacuole called an autophagosome. In studies on yeast, the isolation membrane has been shown to develop from a small vesicle that later transforms into a cup-like structure surrounding the material to be degraded [5]. The formation of an autophagosome (sequestration) is complete when the edges of the 'cup' merge. It has been found that the proteins forming the isolation membrane in yeast are unique, different from those in other cellular compartments, which suggests a de novo formation of this membrane [6]. It is still discussed whether the isolation membrane also forms de novo in higher organisms, including mammals, or if it originates from another organelle, such as endoplasmic reticulum, lysosome or Golgi complex. The sequestration membrane that later gives rise to the autophagosome has been termed phagophore or pre-autophagosome [7]. In yeast and mammalian cells, autophagy occurs at a basal level. The general diameter of autophagosomes is 300-900 nm, and the average level is 500 nm. Since the beginning of the formation of the autophagosomes, cytoplasm and nucleoplasm become darker, but the nucleus structure has no noticeable changes. Mitochondria and endoplasmic reticulum swell, Gorky body expands, and then the membrane-specialized structures such as microvilli disappear, membrane foamed and retracted. At the later stages of autophagy, the volume and number of autophagosomes filled with myelin or liquid increase, and then some gray ingredients and a small number of condensated nuclear materials will exist. These features can be used as morphological indicators during inspection.

Depending on the different ways cellular material is transported to lysosomes, there are three types of autophagy: microautophagy, macroautophagy, chaperone-mediated autophagy (CMA). Macroautophagy is commonly referred to as autophagy, and the cytoplasm is wrapped by the dropped bilayers from the non-ribosomal region of endoplasmic reticulum, the Golgi apparatus and other bilayers. In microautophagy, it also goes through the same process of wrapping, but the substrate is engulfed by inward invagination of the lysosomal membrane. In the process of CMA, intracytoplasmic proteins are bound to the molecular chaperone, then transported to the lysosome cavity, and digested by the lysosomal enzyme. CMA sequester proteins that expose a KFERQ-like pentapeptide which are mediated by heat shock cognate 70 (HSC70) and its co-chaperones. Lysosomal-associated membrane protein 2 (LAMP-2A) acts as a receptor on the lysosome and mediates the degradation of unfolded proteins. Macroautophagy is the major regulated cellular pathway for degrading long-lived proteins and the only known pathway for degrading cytoplasmic organelles (Figure 1). Therefore, this chapter focuses on macroautophagy.

3. Signaling regulation of autophagy

Autophagy is highly conservative during the evolution process. Homologous gene participation in autophagy not only be found in yeasts and Drosophila melanogaster but also in vertebrates and humans. In order to unify the standard, Klionsky, in 2003, named these homologous genes as autophagy-related genes (Atg) to stand for autophagy genes and the corresponding proteins [8]. So far, scientists have already found more than 30 Atgs and most of their homologous analogues. In addition, the Atg protein can be divided into five groups: Atg1 protein kinase complex, Atg9, the class III phosphatidylinositol 3-kinase (PI3K)-Beclin1complex, Atg12 conjugation system and Atg8 conjugation system. Atg1 protein kinase complex is essential for the induction of autophagy. There are two mammalian homologs of Atg1 that appear to function in autophagy, the Unc-51-like kinase 1 (ULK1) and -2 (ULK2), which is the mammalian homologues of serine/threonine protein kinase Atg1, existing in the form of ULK1-mammalian Atg13 (mAtg13) -focal adhesion kinase family interacting protein of 200 kDa (FIP200) -Atg10 complex [9]. Under nutritional deficiency conditions, ULK1 is activated and then phosphorylates mAtg13, FIP200 and itself to initiate autophagy. Regarding the substrates of the Atg1 kinase during autophagy, it is suggested that mAtg13 and FIP200 are phosphorylated by ULKs, and ULKs also undergo autophosphorylation, which is conducive to a conformational change and autophagy induction. Mammalian target of rapammycin (mTOR) can phosphorylate and inactivate ULKs and Atg13 under nutrient-rich conditions. Upon mTOR inhibition by starvation or rapamycin, ULK1 and ULK2 are activated and phosphorylate Atg13 and FIP200, which are essential for autophagy activity. Recent studies have suggested that Atg13 may be phosphorylated by TOR or Atg1/ULKs on different residues [10]. It is likely that phosphorylation of Atg13 is dependent to a greater extent on TOR in yeast, but on Atg1 in Drosophila.

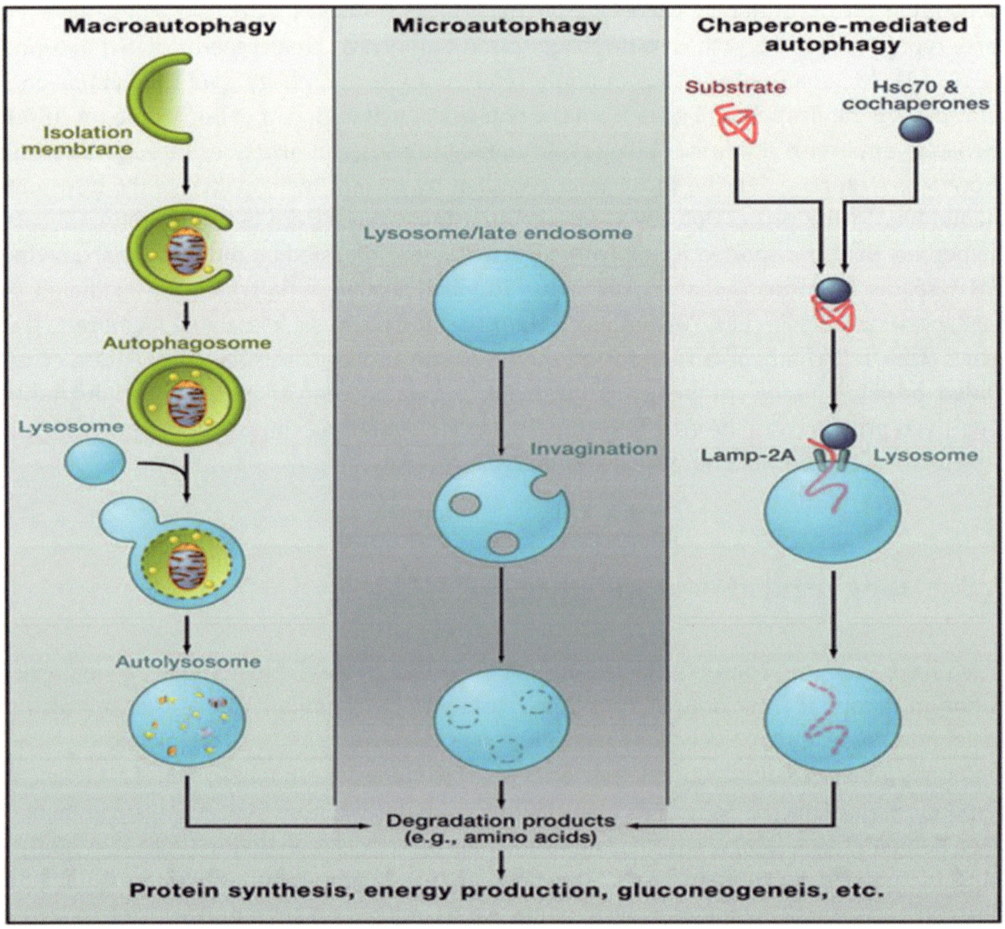

Figure 1. Different Types of Autophagy (Cite from < Mizushima N, Komatsu M. Cell 2011;147(4) 728-741>).

The conjugation of Atg12 and Atg8 is essential for the formation of autophagosomes. Atg12 was the first ubiquitin-like Atg protein to be identified, which can be activated by Atg7 and Atg10. Then it is conjugated to Atg5 and promotes the formation of the autophagy precursor [11]. The amino-acid sequence of Atg12 ends with a glycine residue and there is no protease involved in Atg12 conjugation. Analogous to ubiquitination, there is an E1-like enzyme, Atg7, and Atg12 is activated by forming a thioester bond between the C-terminal Gly 186 of Atg12 and the Cys 507 of Atg7. After activation, Atg12 is transferred to Atg10, which is an E2 enzyme, and is eventually conjugated to the target protein Atg5 at Lys 149 through an isopeptide bond. There is no typical E3 enzyme involved in Atg12-Atg5 conjugation. Atg5 interacts further with a small coiled-coil protein, Atg16, and Atg12-Atg5-Atg16 forms a mul-

http://dx.doi.org/10.5772/53442

timeric complex through the homo-oligomerization of Atg16. The ubiquitin-like (Ubl) protein Atg8 is attached to phosphatidylethanolamine (PE). The C-terminal Arg 117 residue of Atg8 is initially proteolytically removed by a cysteine protease, Atg4, to expose Gly 116. This exposed glycine forms a thioester bond with Cys 507 of Atg7, which is also the site that participates in the Atg12-Atg5 conjugation. This feature differentiates Atg7 from most other E1 enzymes, which activate single Ubl proteins. Activated Atg8 is then transferred to the E2-like enzyme Atg3, also through a thioester bond. In the final step of Atg8 lipidation, Gly 116 of Atg8 is conjugated to PE through an amide bond; Atg8-PE exists in a tightly membrane-associated form. Microtubule-associated protein 1 light chain 3 (LC3) is the mammalian homologues of Atg8. LC3 is activated by Atg7, transferred to Atg3, and conjugated to phosphatidylethanolamine (PE) on the surface of autophagic vacuoles membranes to promote the forming of autophagosomes [12].

Recently, the PI3K-Becline 1 complex and Atg9 have been shown to be the essential components involved in autophagy signaling and the membrane transportation of autophagic vacuoles. This autophagy-specific class III-PI3K-Becline 1 complex appears to be essential to recruit the Atg12-Atg5 conjugation to the pre-autophagosomal structure. Atg12-Atg5 conjugation is then required for the elongation of the isolation membrane and for the proper localization of conjugated LC3/Atg8 [13]. Atg9 is required for autophagy in both yeast and mammalian cells and has been speculated to be involved in delivery of membrane lipids to form autophagosomes. In mammalian cells, mAtg9 traffics between the trans-Golgi network, endosomes and newly formed autophagosomes [14].

Cells regulate autophagy through a set of precise signaling pathways including integrating nutriment, growth factors, hormones, stress and intracellular energy information. A key regulator point of autophagy in mammals is kinase mTOR. The kinase TOR is a major evolutionarily conserved sensor in the autophagy signaling pathway in eukaryotes, but it also regulates many other aspects of cell function, including transcription, translation, and cell size and cytoskeletal organization. In mammals, mTOR can be included in two different complexes, mTORC1 and mTORC2. Although these two TOR complexes share common components, they display distinct cellular functions and phosphorylate different downstream substrates. The activity of mTORC1 is regulated via the integration of many signals, including growth factors, insulin, nutrients, energy availability, and cell stressors such as hypoxia, osmotic stress, reactive oxygen species (ROS) and viral infection. mTORC1 is the only known target of the drug rapamycin and is required for signaling to ribosomal S6 kinases (S6K) and eIF4E-binding proteins (4EBP1 and 4EBP2). mTORC1 has recently been shown to consist of four proteins: mTOR, mLST8 (also known as GbL), proline-rich PKB/Akt substrate 40-kDa (PRAS40), and raptor (regulatory associated protein of mTOR); and it plays a major role in controlling translation and cell growth in response to nutrients. The adaptor protein is common to both mTOR complexes. Raptor binds mTOR, S6K and 4EBP1/2 and facilitates mTOR phosphorylation of these molecules; but whether raptor enhances or represses mTOR kinase activity remains unclear [15]. Unlike mTORC1, mTORC2 has some functions that cannot be inhibited by rapamycin, including the control of actin cytoskeleton dynamics. The mTORC2 complex consists of mTOR, mLST8, mammalian stress-activated protein kinase-interacting protein 1 (mSin1), and rapamycin-insensitive companion of mTOR (rictor). Recent studies indicate that when eutrophy, mTOR activates the PI3K-I/ protein kinase B (PKB) signaling pathway, it leads multiple serine sites to phosphorylation and then reduces the affinity of Atg13 and Atg1. Since Atg1-Atg13 compounds decreased, Atg9 cannot be transferred to the autophagosome formation sites and autophagy was inhibited.

AMP-activated protein kinase (AMPK) was initially identified as a serine/threonine kinase that negatively regulates several key enzymes of the lipid anabolism. Meanwhile, AMPK is regarded as the major energy-sensing kinase that activates a whole variety of catabolic processes in multicellular organisms such as glucose uptake and metabolism, while simultaneously inhibiting several anabolic pathways, such as lipid, protein, and carbohydrate biosynthesis. Activated AMPK can inhibit mTOR by interfering with the activity of GTPase Rheb and with protein synthesis, degrade the phosphorylation of ULK1 and promote disintegration of ULK1 from the mTOR compounds. In starved cells, when the AMP/ATP ratio increases; the binding of AMP to AMPK promotes its activation by the AMPK kinase LKB. Moreover, Ca^{2+}/calmodulin-dependent kinase kinase beta (CaMKK-beta) has been identified as being an AMPK kinase. The activity of AMPK is required for autophagy to be induced in response to starvation in mammalian cells and in yeast in a TORC1-dependent manner. Moreover, autophagy induction is also dependent on the inhibition of mTORC1 by AMPK in non-starved cells in response to an increase in free cytosolic Ca^{2+}. In this setting, the activation of AMPK and stimulation of autophagy are dependent on CaMKK-beta. The induction of autophagy through AMPK activation probably also occurs in other settings, such as hypoxia. AMPK is probably a general regulator of autophagy upstream of mTOR [16]. Another potential candidate of autophagy regulation down-stream of AMPK is elongation factor-2 kinase (eEF-2 kinase), which controls the rate of peptide elongation [17]. Activation of eEF-2 kinase increases autophagy and slows protein translation. The activity of eEF-2 kinase is regulated by mTOR, S6K, and AMPK. During periods of ATP depletion, AMPK is activated and eEF-2 kinase is phosphorylated, leading to a balance between the inhibition of peptide elongation and the induction of autophagy. However, how eEF-2 kinase impinges on the molecular machinery of autophagy remains to be elucidated.

There also is an indirectly-TOR-dependent signaling pathway, named class I PI3K/Akt pathway, which when responding to insulin-like and other growth factor signals, the signaling molecules link receptor tyrosine kinases to activate TOR kinase and thereby repress autophagy. In addition, autophagy can mediate inactive proteins to degrade to amino acids and then provide metabolic substrates for cardiac development and ischemic hypoxia forming a cardiac protection method. Autophagy is among the important mechanisms of hypoxic adaptation and is perhaps one of the last resorts for the salvage of ATP in hypoxic cells and organs.

p53 is a responsive stress protein which also plays a crucial role in the regulation of autophagy through the transcription-dependent/independent pathways. In the transcription-independent pathway, p53 can activate AMPK and down-regulate mTOR; in the transcription-dependent pathway, through the up-regulation of PTEN (inhibitor of mTOR), the tuberous sclerosis-1 (TSC1) gene or cell death gene damage-regulated autophagy modulator 1 (DRAM1), mTOR is down-regulated, and autophagy is induced (Figure 2). In addition, c-jun N signal kinases (JNK), GTPases, Erk1/2, ceramide are also involved in regulating autophagy. The cytoplasmic form of p53 has been shown to have an inhibitory effect on autophagy, suggesting that activation of autophagy by p53 depends on its transactivating effect on genes such as DRAM1 [18].

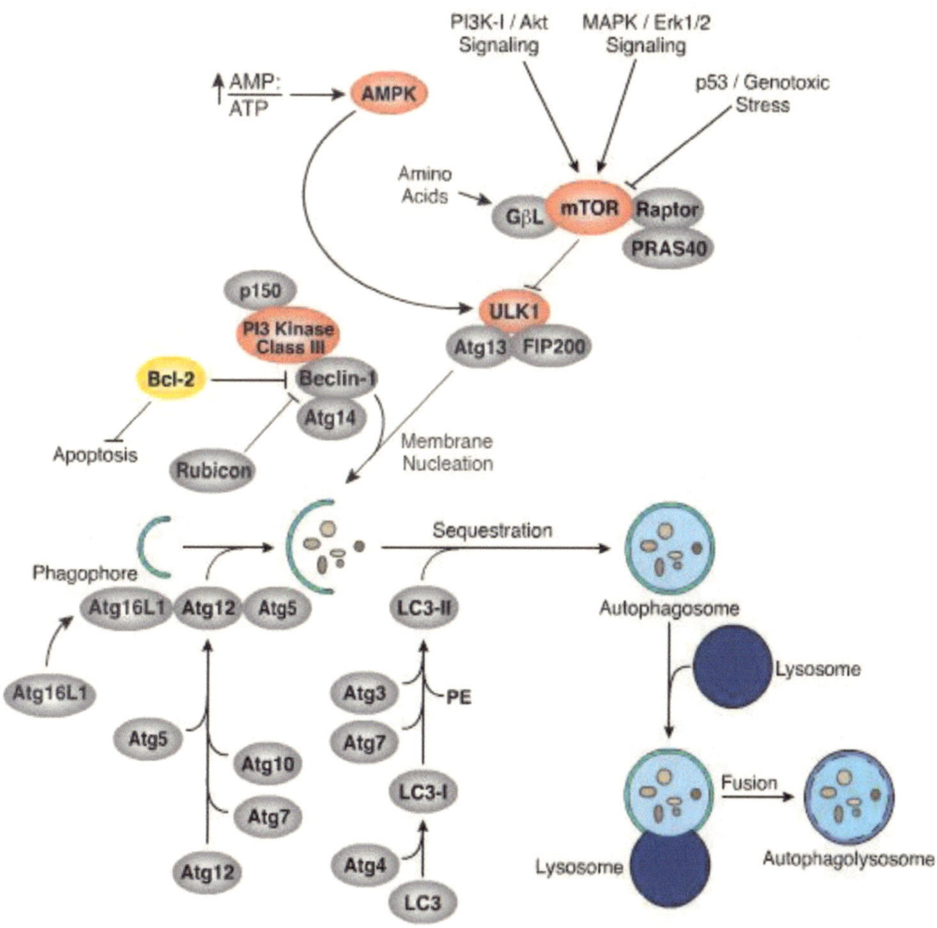

Figure 2. Signaling Pathway of Autophagy (Cite from http://www.cellsignal.com/).

4. The role of autophagy in the maintenance of normal myocardium

In the basal state, autophagy showed low expression in the heart to maintain normal myocardial function. And most of its function is to perform homeostatic functions by eliminating long-live organelles and proteins. Autophagy can be upregulated rapidly when myocardium cells need to generate intracellular nutrients and energy, for example during starvation or trophic factor withdrawal. Nutritional status, hormonal factors, and other cues like temperature, oxygen concentrations, and cell density are important in the control of autophagy.

The molecular mechanism of autophagy is still poorly understood. There are more than 30 genes that have been confirmed to be related to autophagy, and half of them are highly conservative in most metazoa [19]. Knockout Atg5 gene (a decisive gene in autophagy) in early stage adult rat hearts has showed no obvious abnormality, however, after increased afterload for one week, left ventricular can cause myocardial ubiquitination and mitochondrial aggregation, resulting in myocardial hypertrophy and decrease in myocardial contractility, which indicates that autophagy may play an important role in maintenance of homeostasis, size of myocardium, general construction and function of myocardial cells. Paradoxically, partially reduced autophagic activity caused by heterozygous deletion of Beclin 1 improves cardiac function upon pressure overload. Consistent with this phenomenon, partial suppression of autophagy with histone deacetylase (HDAC) inhibitors can ameliorate pressure overload-induced cardiac hypertrophy in mice [20]. These data suggest that partial, but not complete, suppression of autophagy may be beneficial.

In short, autophagy adapts to the myocardial energy demand by maintaining energy metabolism, so as to protect the myocardial function.

5. The protective effect of autophagy in myocardial ischemia/hypoxia

In recent years, a large number of studies suggested that autophagy played a protective role to rescue cardiomyocytes in ischemia/hypoxia. In [21], researchers discovered that 40 mins of hypoxia induced significant autophagosome and autolysosome formation, according to a rabbit hypoxic heart model. At the same time, ultrastructural analysis revealed autophagosomes in close proximity to swollen and fragmented mitochondria. And in rodents, 30 mins after ischemia induced dramatic up-regulation of autophagosome formation [22]. Previous report also demonstrated that the level of autophagy was rapidly increased within 30 mins after coronary ligation in mice, especially in the risk area (salvaged cardiomyocytes bordering the infarcted area) [23]. Recent work has revealed that inactivation of hypoxia-inducible factor 1α (HIF-1α) in fibroblasts blunts hypoxia-induced autophagy [24]. These results strongly suggested that autophagy was activated by myocardial ischemia/hypoxia. Furthermore, these investigators reported that suppression of autophagy using 3-methyladenine or bafilomycin A1 enhanced myocyte death triggered by glucose deprivation. During postinfarction cardiac remodeling, lysosomes and autophagosomes became more numerous in the cardiomyocytes, thus ensuring that autophagy could provide enough energy to cardiomyocytes. The protective effects of autophagy may be that cells were likely to be provided energy, free amino acids and fatty acids through decomposition of their own material.

Additionally, autophagy may maintain cardiomyocyte survival after ischemia/hypoxia by inhibiting apoptosis [25]. Autophagy is a recycling process of cytoplasmic components, such as long-lived proteins and organelles. The prosurvival role of autophagy has been observed in yeast, plants, flies, and mammals. Inhibition of autophagy results in accumulation of cytoplasmic components and promotion of apoptosis. Treatment with pharmacological autophagy inhibitors and knockdown of Atg genes (Atg5, Atg10, Atg12, and Beclin 1) can increase apoptosis and cell death in nutrient-deprived cells. In reference [26], autophagy delayed apoptotic cell death in breast cancer cells following DNA damage. These results suggested that the effect of inhibiting apoptosis may be related to autophagosomes wrapping damaged mitochondria, because it will not only prevent the release of cytochrome C, but also inhibit the formation of apoptotic bodies.

Numerous studies show that mTOR is a key factor in regulating autophagy in ischemia/hypoxia. In mammalian cells, phosphorylation of mTOR inhibits cell autophagy. Conversely, dephosphorylation of mTOR enhances autophagy. The activity of mTOR is adjusted by many factors. AMPK is the important factor which would inhibit the activity of mTOR to enhance autophagy in ischemia. AMPK serves as a general integrator of metabolic responses to changes in energy availability and is activated in response to elevations of the AMP/ATP ratio. Data in reference [27] suggested that autophagy has been reported to be up-regulated in response to reduced cellular content of ATP. In cultured cardiac myocytes, glucose deprivation caused significant reduction in the levels of ATP, which coincided with up-regulation of autophagy. Moreover, myocardial ischemia causes a decrease in ATP levels and an increase in the AMP/ATP ratio, resulting in activation of the AMPK [28]. Under conditions of stress (including hypoxia and ischemia), a signaling cascade is initiated involving phosphorylation of AMPK and subsequent inhibition of mTOR. Inhibition of mTOR, in concert with other protein partners, provides the critical step in initiating autophagosome formation.

6. The expression and regulation of autophagy during myocardial ischemia/reperfusion

Autophagy is induced during myocardial ischemia. Although it was speculated that activation of autophagy may be reverted when ischemia is relieved, in fact, autophagy may be further enhanced by reperfusion [22, 29]. A variety of factors that can regulate the autophagy during myocardial ischemia/reperfusion, such as ROS generated by mitochondrial respiration, endoplasmic reticulum stress, calcium, vitamin D compounds, ATP, thapsigargin, calcium protease, and so on. Different signal transduction pathways are involved in the occurrence of autophagy at different stages of myocardial ischemia/reperfusion.

6.1. The role of Beclin 1 in the occurrence of autophagy during myocardial ischemia/reperfusion

Induction of autophagy in the ischemic phase was accompanied by activation of AMPK and mTOR. In contrast, autophagy during reperfusion was accompanied by upregulation of Beclin 1 rather than by activation of AMPK. Induction of autophagy and cardiac injury during the reperfusion phase was significantly attenuated in Beclin 1+/- mice. Collectively, in the ischemic heart, autophagy is stimulated through an AMPK-dependent mechanism, whereas ischemia/reperfusion stimulates autophagy through a Beclin 1-dependent but not an AMPK-independent pathway [22]. Using cultured cardiomyocytes, previous studies have demonstrated that the inhibition of autophagy by urocortin during the reperfusion phase is mediated in part by inhibition of Beclin 1 expression, an effect which is mediated by activation of the PI3K/Akt pathway [30]. Recent experimental data also show that the clearance of autophagosomes is impaired in myocardial reperfusion injury which is mediated in part by ROS-induced decline in LAMP-2A and upregulation of Beclin 1, contributing to increased cardiomyocyte death [31, 32]. Thus, ROS and ROS-mediated upregulation of Beclin 1 in the myocardial reperfusion phase may play an important role in the occurrence of autophagy. Therefore, it is now widely recognized that the autophagy was induced through the AMPK-eEF2K/mTOR pathway during the ischemic phase of ischemic/reperfusion injury, but was triggered through the Class III PI3K/Beclin 1 pathway during the reperfusion phase.

6.2. The role of Bcl-2 family members in the occurrence of autophagy during myocardial ischemia/reperfusion

It is well known that the Bcl-2 family proteins play essential roles in regulating apoptosis in the cardiovascular system, and several studies have revealed that the Bcl-2 family members (Bnip3, Bcl-2, Bcl-XL, Bax, etc.) also play important roles in the induction of autophagy during myocardial ischemia/reperfusion injury.

6.2.1. Bnip3

Bnip3 (Bcl-2/adenovirus E1B-19 KD interacting protein 3) with a single Bcl-2 homology 3 (BH3) domain is a pro-apoptotic Bcl-2 family protein which is most sensitive to hypoxia and plays an important role in myocardial ischemia/reperfusion injury. It was found that the overexpression of Bnip3 significantly increased autophagy, whereas, overexpression of the dominant-negative Bnip3 significantly reduced autophagy induced by myocardial ischemia/reperfusion in HL-1 cardiac myocytes [33]. These results suggest that Bnip3 plays a fundamental role in the induction of autophagy during myocardial ischemia and reperfusion. However, more studies are still needed to clarify the role of Bnip3 in response to ischemia/reperfusion, and the most reasonable explanation is that the mitochondrial dysfunction caused by Bnip3 can enhance the level of autophagy in order to remove damaged organelles.

6.2.2. Bcl-2/Bcl-XL and Bax

Bcl-2 family members are key modulators of apoptosis that have recently been shown to also regulate autophagy. Transgenic mice overexpressing the anti-apoptotic human Bcl-2 cDNA in the heart is effective at reducing myocardial reperfusion injury and improving heart function [34, 35]. However, blockage of the activity of the proapoptotic molecule Bax in a knockout mouse model attenuates ischemia/reperfusion injury [36]. Recent reports demonstrated that Beclin 1 possessed a BH3 domain. The BH3 domain of Beclin 1 is bound to and inhibited by Bcl-2 or Bcl-XL [37, 38]. A BH3 mutant of Beclin1 which has reduced affinity for Bcl-XL/Bcl-2 was a more potent inducer of autophagy than wild type Beclin 1. Overexpression of Bcl-2 in the heart reduced starvation-induced autophagy. Thus, Bcl-2 not only functions as an antiapoptotic protein, but also as an antiautophagy protein via its inhibitory interaction with Beclin 1. These antiapoptosis and antiautophagy functions of Bcl-2 may protect the myocardium against ischemia/reperfusion injury [39]. Meanwhile, some studies found that Bnip3 enhanced autophagy, possibly due to competitive disruption of Bcl-2 binding to Beclin 1 [24] or interacting with Rheb to inhibit mTOR [40]. Of course, more studies are needed to clarify these relationships.

6.3. The role of angiotensin II (Ang II) receptor signaling in the induction of autophagy during myocardial ischemia/reperfusion

Recent report demonstrated that overexpression of Ang II type 1 (AT1) receptor caused a significant increase in autophagy after treatment with Ang II in cultured neonatal rat cardiomyocytes. However, overexpression of the Ang II type 2 (AT2) receptor can inhibit autophagy in an Ang II-independent manner. Neonatal cardiomyocytes cultured from hypertrophic heart rats (HHRs) were more susceptible to AT1 receptor-stimulated autophagy than cardiomyocytes from normal heart rats (NHRs). Moreover, there was a greater up-regulation of autophagic markers in adult HHR hearts than in NHR hearts following ischemia/reperfusion in vitro [41]. Additionally, AT1 receptor blockaded with olmesartan plays a protective role in myocardial ischemia-reperfusion injury [42]. Therefore, it is inferred that Ang II/AT1 receptor signaling might also be involved in the stimulation of autophagy during myocardial ischemia/reperfusion.

Thus, in addition to the Beclin 1, many Bcl-2 family members and angiotensin II/AT1 receptor signaling may also be involved in the stimulation of autophagy, but additional studies are needed to clarify the role of these pathways in the occurrence of autophagy during ischemia/reperfusion injury of the heart.

7. The role of autophagy in myocardial ischemia/reperfusion

The autophagy is induced during the ischemia/reperfusion process; however, the role of autophagy during myocardial ischemia/reperfusion is still inconclusive.

It is well-documented that autophagy occurs at basal levels but can be further induced by stresses, such as nutrient depletion. Autolysosomal degradation of membrane lipids and proteins generate free fatty acids and amino acids, which can be reused to maintain mitochondrial ATP production and protein synthesis and promote cell survival. When the myocardium was suppressed with ischemia, the blood supply was decreased and the energy was insufficient, which means that there was an inadequate supply of nutrients. In these conditions, AMPK acts as a sensor for energy deprivation and activation of AMPK mediates metabolic adaptation during ischemia.

Many studies have shown that the autophagy induced by lack of blood supply plays a protective effect during periods of ischemia. For example, see [43], autophagy is significantly up-regulated during chronic ischemia in the pig heart. In this model, the level of autophagy was inversely correlated with that of apoptosis in the ischemic area. The ischemic area was recovered when the coronary flow was restored, suggesting that autophagy may protect myocardium from apoptosis during hibernation. Inhibition of endogenous AMPK suppressed autophagy during prolonged ischemia, which was accompanied by enlargement of the myocardial infarction. Although one may speculate that activation of autophagy may be reverted as soon as ischemia is relieved, the level of autophagy in fact further increases during reperfusion. However, a higher level of autophagy is not due to the lack of energy during blood flow restoration after reperfusion. Mechanisms mediating autophagy during reperfusion appear different from those involved in autophagy during ischemia. Energy crisis, a major stimulus for autophagy, in the heart is at least partially resolved at the time of reperfusion [32]. Instead, ROS appears to be a major promoter of autophagy during reperfusion. ROS induces mitochondrial damage, as evidenced by mitochondrial permeability transition pore (mPTP) opening and mitochondrial fragmentation, which in turn promotes autophagy and/or mitophagy, a specialized form of autophagy which removes mitochondria [44]. ROS oxidizes and inhibits the cysteine protease activity of Atg4, which results in LC3 lipidation and autophagy.

Whether autophagy induced during reperfusion is beneficial or detrimental remains controversial. Previous data [32] have shown that, although autophagic flux is inhibited during ischemia/reperfusion, enhancing autophagic flux during ischemia/reperfusion protects against ischemia/reperfusion injury in cardiomyocytes in vitro. The number of Bax (+) cardiac cells induced by reperfusion was significantly increased when Beclin-1 or Atg-5 were knocked out, but was reduced when there was an overexpression of Beclin-1 [45]. In an in vivo model of myocardial ischemia/reperfusion in pigs, autophagy was significantly activated when the coronary perfusion is restored, which was accompanied by reduction of apoptosis in myocardial cells and almost complete recovery of cardiac function [46]. Other experiments have also demonstrated that autophagy activation during myocardial ischemia/reperfusion can remove the damaged mitochondria caused by Bnip3. These results indicate that autophagy may promote cell survival during myocardial ischemia/reperfusion injury.

In contrast, study in reference [30] showed that inhibiting autophagy by treatment with 3-methyladenine or by Beclin1 knock down increases the survival of cardiomyocytes after ischemia/reperfusion in vitro. As results in [22], the myocardial infarct size increased by 40% in rats subjected to reperfusion, while the infarct size was down-regulated to

http://dx.doi.org/10.5772/53442

20% after the autophagy gene Beclin1 knockout. Inhibition of cathepsin, which can degrade autophagosomes, can significantly reduce myocardial cell damage and apoptosis during the reperfusion phase. Therefore, the roles of autophagy are not very clear during myocardial reperfusion. Further studies are needed to investigate the real roles of autophagy in myocardial ischemia/reperfusion injury. However, it is still speculated that the excessive degradation of important proteins and organelles by autophagy will cause cell death.

8. The role of autophagy in aging hearts subjected to ischemia/reperfusion

Aging is characterized by a progressive accumulation of damaged cells and organs. Autophagy degraded damaged organelles and macromolecule materials in stress, which prolonged life span [47]. Autophagy, including the autophagosome formation, the maturation, and the efficiency of autophagosome-lysosome fusion, as well as the proteolysis activity of lysosomes, declines with age [48]. All of these factors induce an abundance of the lipofuscin polymer accumulated in lysosomes. The lipofuscin polymer could not be degraded by lysosomes. The lysosome with an abundance of lipofuscin polymer lost its bio-function. Therefore, some damaged organelles and macromolecule materials could not be cleaned up, which accounted for the aging process. Several studies supported enhancing autophagy as the most efficient anti-aging intervention [49, 50].

In the heart, autophagy maintains a low basal level to perform biological functions, such as degrading dysfunctional organelles, maintaining cardiac morphology and function [51, 52]. However, autophagy in cardiomyocytes were up-regulated in response to environmental stress conditions, such as ATP depletion (e.g. during starvation), oxidative damage, and mitochondrial permeability transition pore opening (e.g. myocardial ischemia/reperfusion injury) [53, 54]. Activation of autophagy during ischemia is essential for cell survival and maintenance of cardiac function. However, autophagy was activated in the heart subjected to ischemia/reperfusion. Recent reviews show autophagy during reperfusion could be either protective or detrimental [41]. Serious induction of autophagy accompanied by robust up-regulation of Beclin-1 could cause autophagic cell death, thereby proving to be detrimental. If ischemia is mild, activation of autophagy during reperfusion may be modest and thus may not be harmful.

Until now, there is little information related to autophagy in myocardial ischemia/reperfusion injury in aging. Our primary data showed that ischemia/reperfusion injury was more serious in aging hearts compared with young hearts. Beclin-1 was increased in aging hearts subjected to ischemia/reperfusion, which indicated activated autophagy. However, further research is needed to know the exact role of autophagy in myocardial ischemia/reperfusion injury, especially in aging. Moreover, recent studies suggest that autophagy is one of the important mechanisms in myocardial ischemia/reperfusion preconditioning. Decreased autophagy may contribute to the weakened protective role of preconditioning in aging hearts subjected to ischemia/reperfusion. Therefore, excessive autophagy results in autophagic cell death and loss of cardiomyocytes, responsible for the worsening of aging myocardial ischemia/reperfusion injury. The molecular transduction pathways need to be investigated further. It could help to develop therapies that up-regulate the repair qualities of the autophagic process and down-regulate the cell death aspects, which would be of great value in the treatment of aging myocardial ischemia/reperfusion injury.

9. The investigative methods of autophagy

9.1. Electron microscopy

Electron microscopy is the most reliable method for testing autophagy at present and can be used to quantify the autophagic activity of cells. In electron microscopy, the autophagosome is composed of double membrane structures that wrap abnormal cytoplasmic material. Then, the autolysosome is composed of the monolayer membrane structure which wraps cytoplasm ingredients at different degradation stages. Because of the difficulty of distinguishing between autophagosomes and autolysosomes, both of them are often called 'autophagic vacuoles'. The proportion of autophagic vacuoles is calcultaed accounting for the total area or volume of cytoplasm through electron microscopy, which can be used to quantify cell autophagic activity.

9.2. Specific markers

Atg8 includes three kinds of homology in humans: GABARAP, GATE-16 and LC3. The C-terminal proteolysis of LC3 is processed by Atg4, based on the residues Phe80 and Leu82 of LC3 that may be recognized by Atg4, and immediately follows synthesis to yield a soluble form, LC3-I. LC3-I is converted to a membrane bound form, LC3-II, through a ubiquitin-like reaction involving Atg7, a ubiquitin-acivating enzyme (E1)-like enzyme, and Atg3, a ubiquitin-conjugating enzyme (E1)-like enzyme (E2). LC3-II combines to phosphatidyl ethanolamine (PE) on the membrane surface of autophagic vacuoles. In addition, LC3-II is easily located within the cell after the formation of the fusion protein with the green fluorescent protein (GFP). Therefore, GFP-LC3 II is usually used as the marker protein of the autophagosome membrane in mammalian cells.

Beclin 1 is involved in the formation of autophagosomes, which are the mammalian yeast homologues of Apg6/Vps30. Some researches show that autophagy is significantly attenuated in Beclin 1+/- mice, but apoptosis is normal. These results indicate that Beclin 1 is a significant positive control gene in autophagy. Therefore, by testing the expression level of Beclin1, combined with other biochemistry indexes, the autophagic activity of cells can be monitored and judged dynamically.

9.3. Monodansylcadaverine (MDC) dyeing

MDC is a kind of fluorescent dye, which is used as a tracer of the autophagic vacuoles. MDC can specifically bind to the ubiquitin-proteasome sample protein binding systems (Atg8). In addition, MDC can be absorbed by cells and selectively gathered in autophagic vesicles, showing punctuate structure under fluorescence microscope. Therefore, the quantitative detection of autophagy uses this method. However, most of the MDC is not marked in GFP-LC3. However, MDC is not a reliable marker of autophagosomes. Therefore, other experimental evidences that represent the autophagic activity of cells are needed.

9.4. Specific agonists and inhibitors

Rapamycin is a novel macrolide immunosuppressant, and induces cell autophagy by inhibiting the mTOR pathway. In scientific studies, Rapamycin is the specific agonist of autophagy. The main inhibitors of the phosphor-lipin acid radical inositol 3 kinase include 3-MA, which can specifically block the fusion of autophagic vacuoles and lysosomes. Rapamycin is widely used as an inhibitor of autophagy, and Wortmannin, LY29400297 and Bafilomycin A1 are included.

10. Perspectives

Autophagy is intimately involved not only in the physiology of the heart, but also in development of the ischemic heart. The regulation of autophagy may be a new approach for the treatment of ischemic heart disease. However, to translate the knowledge of autophagy into treatment of ischemic heart disease, it is necessary to know more precisely about the formation, function, mechanism, and regulation of autophagy. When autophagy is protective and when it is detrimental for the ischemic heart needs further clarification. Another problem is how to regulate autophagy without affecting other life activities, since even the evolutionarily conserved autophagy genes also have autophagy-dependent functions. There is continuing research on this topic. In addition, the signaling mechanisms positively or negatively regulating autophagy in the heart have not been completely elucidated. Judging from the diversity of autophagy regulators, it is believed that more unknown signal transduction pathways will also be proven to be involved in the activation of autophagy. In short, only clarifying the activation mechanism, function, time course, and its relationship with cell death, etc. autophagy can truly benefit patients with ischemic heart disease.

Acknowledgements

This work was supported by the grants from the Natural Sciences Foundation of China (NSFC) 81270283, the NSFC 81070263, the NSFC 30973163, KZ201110025023 from Science and Technology Plan Project of Beijing Municipal Education Commission, and the Funding

Project for Academic Human Resources Development in Institutions of Higher Learning under the Jurisdiction of Beijing Municipality (PHR201106112).

Author details

Suli Zhang[1], Jin Wang[2], Yunhui Du[3], Jianyu Shang[1], Li Wang[2], Jie Wang[2], Ke Wang[1], Kehua Bai[2], Tingting Lv[1], Xiao Li[1] and Huirong Liu[1*]

*Address all correspondence to: liuhr2000@126.com

1 Department of Physiology and Pathophysiology, School of Basic Medical Sciences, Capital Medical University, Beijing, P.R. China

2 Department of Physiology, Shanxi Medical University, Taiyuan, Shanxi, P.R. China

3 Department of Biochemistry and Molecular Biology, Marine College, Shandong Medical University, Weihai, Shandong, P.R. China

References

[1] Ashford TP, Porter KR. Cytoplasmic components in hepatic cell lysosomes. J Cell Biol 1962;12(1) 198–202.

[2] Klionsky DJ. Autophagy revisited: a conversation with Christian de Duve. Autophagy 2008;4(6) 740-743.

[3] Levine B, Klionsky DJ. Development by self-digestion: molecular mechanisms and biological functions of autophagy. Dev Cell 2004;6(4) 463-477.

[4] Levine B, Yuan J. Autophagy in cell death: an innocent convict? J Clin Invest 2005;115(10) 2679-2688.

[5] Sneve ML, Øverbye A, Fengsrud M, Seglen PO. Comigration of two autophagosome-associated dehydrogenases on two-dimensional polyacrylamide gels. Autophagy 2005;1(3) 157-1562.

[6] Noda T, Suzuki K, Ohsumi Y. Yeast autophagosomes: de novo formation of a membrane structure. Trends Cell Biol 2002;12(5) 231-235.

[7] Tanida I, Ueno T, Kominami E. LC3 conjugation system in mammalian autophagy. Int J Biochem Cell Biol 2004;36(12) 2503-2518.

[8] Klionsky DJ, Cregg JM, Dunn WA Jr, Emr SD, Sakai Y, Sandoval IV, Sibirny A, Subramani S, Thumm M, Veenhuis M, Ohsumi Y. A unified nomenclature for yeast autophagy-related genes. Dev Cell 2003;5(4) 539-545.

[9] Cheong H, Lindsten T, Thompson CB. Autophagy and ammonia. Autophagy 2012;8(1) 122-123.

[10] Ganley IG, Lam du H, Wang J, Ding X, Chen S, Jiang X. ULK1.ATG13.FIP200 complex mediates mTOR signaling and is essential for autophagy. J Biol Chem 2009;284(18) 12297-12305.

[11] Yamaguchi M, Noda NN, Yamamoto H, Shima T, Kumeta H, Kobashigawa Y, Akada R, Ohsumi Y, Inagaki F. Structural insights into atg10-mediated formation of the autophagy-essential atg12-atg5 conjugate. Structure 2012;20(7) 1244-1254.

[12] Mizushima N, Yoshimori T. How to interpret LC3 immunoblotting. Autophagy 2007;3(6) 542-545.

[13] Shpilka T, Weidberg H, Pietrokovski S, Elazar Z. Atg8: an autophagy-related ubiquitin-like protein family. Genome Biol 2011;12(7) 226.

[14] Webber JL, Tooze SA. New insights into the function of Atg9. FEBS Lett 2010;584(7) 1319-1326.

[15] Distefano G, Boca M, Rowe I, Wodarczyk C, Ma L, Piontek KB, Germino GG, Pandolfi PP, Boletta A. Polycystin-1 regulates extracellular signal-regulated kinase-dependent phosphorylation of tuberin to control cell size through mTOR and its downstream effectors S6K and 4EBP1. Mol Cell Biol 2009;29(9) 2359-2371

[16] Pfisterer SG, Mauthe M, Codogno P, Proikas-Cezanne T. Ca2+/calmodulin-dependent kinase (CaMK) signaling via CaMKI and AMP-activated protein kinase contributes to the regulation of WIPI-1 at the onset of autophagy. Mol Pharmacol 2011;80(6) 1066-1075.

[17] Browne GJ, Finn SG, Proud CG. Stimulation of the AMP-activated protein kinase leads to activation of eukaryotic elongation factor 2 kinase and to its phosphorylation at a novel site, serine 398. J Biol Chem 2004;279(13) 12220-12231.

[18] Zhang XD, Qin ZH, Wang J. The role of p53 in cell metabolism. Acta Pharmacol Sin 2010;31(9) 1208-1212.

[19] Yorimitsu T, Klionsky DJ. Autophagy: molecular machinery for self-eating. Cell Death Differ 2005;12(Suppl 2) 1542-1552.

[20] Cao DJ, Wang ZV, Battiprolu PK, Jiang N, Morales CR, Kong Y, Rothermel BA, Gillette TG, Hill JA. Histone deacetylase (HDAC) inhibitors attenuate cardiac hypertrophy by suppressing autophagy. Proc Natl Acad Sci U S A 2011;108(10) 4123-4128.

[21] Decker R.S, Wildenthal K. Lysosomal alterations in hypoxic and reoxygenated hearts. I. Ultrastructural and cytochemical changes. Am. J. Pathol 1980;98(2) 425-444.

[22] Matsui Y, Takagi H, Qu X, Abdellatif M, Sakoda H, Asano T, Levine B, Sadoshima J. Distinct roles of autophagy in the heart during ischemia and reperfusion: roles of AMP-activated protein kinase and Beclin 1 in mediating autophagy. Circ. Res 2007;100(6) 914-922.

[23] Kanamori H, Takemura G, Goto K, Maruyama R, Ono K, Nagao K, Tsujimoto A, Ogino A, Takeyama T, Kawaguchi T, Watanabe T, Kawasaki M, Fujiwara T, Fujiwara H, Seishima M, Minatoguchi S. Autophagy limits acute myocardial infarction induced by permanent coronary artery occlusion. Am J Physiol Heart Circ Physiol 2011;300(6) H2261-H2271.

[24] Zhang H, Bosch-Marce M, Shimoda LA, Tan YS, Baek JH, Wesley JB, et al. Mitochondrial autophagy is an HIF-1-dependent adaptive metabolic response to hypoxia. The Journal of biological chemistry 2008;283(16) 10892-10903.

[25] Boya P, Gonzalez-Polo RA, Casares N, Perfettini JL, Dessen P, Larochette N, Metivier D, Meley D, Souquere S, Yoshimori T, Pierron G, Codogno P, Kroemer G. Inhibition of macroautophagy triggers apoptosis. Mol Cell Biol 2005;25(3) 1025-1040.

[26] Abedin MJ, Wang D, McDonnell MA, Lehmann U, Kelekar A. Autophagy delays apoptotic death in breast cancer cells following DNAdamage. Cell Death Differ 2007;14(3) 500-510.

[27] Lum JJ, DeBerardinis RJ, Thompson CB. Autophagy in metazoans: cell survival in the land of plenty. Nat Rev Mol Cell Biol 2005;6(6) 439-448.

[28] Arad M, Seidman CE, Seidman JG. AMP-activated protein kinase in the heart: role during health and disease. Circ Res 2007;100(4) 474-488.

[29] Gurusamy N, Lekli I, Gorbunov NV, Gherghiceanu M, Popescu LM, Das DK. Cardioprotection by adaptation to ischaemia augments autophagy in association with BAG-1 protein. Journal of cellular and molecular medicine 2009;13(2) 373-387.

[30] Valentim L, Laurence KM, Townsend PA, Carroll CJ, Soond S, Scarabelli TM, et al. Urocortin inhibits Beclin1-mediated autophagic cell death in cardiac myocytes exposed to ischaemia/reperfusion injury. Journal of molecular and cellular cardiology 2006;40(6) 846-852.

[31] Ma X, Liu H, Foyil SR, Godar RJ, Weinheimer CJ, Hill JA, et al. Impaired autophagosome clearance contributes to cardiomyocyte death in ischemia/reperfusion injury. Circulation 2012;125(25) 3170-3181.

[32] Hariharan N, Zhai P, Sadoshima J. Oxidative stress stimulates autophagic flux during ischemia/reperfusion. Antioxidants & redox signaling 2011;14(11) 2179-2190.

[33] Hamacher-Brady A, Brady NR, Logue SE, Sayen MR, Jinno M, Kirshenbaum LA, et al. Response to myocardial ischemia/reperfusion injury involves Bnip3 and autophagy. Cell death and differentiation 2007;14(1) 146-157.

[34] Chen Z, Chua CC, Ho YS, Hamdy RC, Chua BH. Overexpression of Bcl-2 attenuates apoptosis and protects against myocardial I/R injury in transgenic mice. American journal of physiology Heart and circulatory physiology 2001;280(5) H2313-H2320.

[35] Imahashi K, Schneider MD, Steenbergen C, Murphy E. Transgenic expression of Bcl-2 modulates energy metabolism, prevents cytosolic acidification during ischemia, and reduces ischemia/reperfusion injury. Circulation research 2004;95(7) 734-741.

[36] Hochhauser E, Kivity S, Offen D, Maulik N, Otani H, Barhum Y, et al. Bax ablation protects against myocardial ischemia-reperfusion injury in transgenic mice. American journal of physiology Heart and circulatory physiology 2003;284(6) H2351-H2359.

[37] Oberstein A, Jeffrey PD, Shi Y. Crystal structure of the Bcl-XL-Beclin 1 peptide complex: Beclin 1 is a novel BH3-only protein. The Journal of biological chemistry 2007;282(17) 13123-13132.

[38] Maiuri MC, Le Toumelin G, Criollo A, Rain JC, Gautier F, Juin P, et al. Functional and physical interaction between Bcl-X(L) and a BH3-like domain in Beclin-1. The EMBO journal 2007;26(10) 2527-2539.

[39] Pattingre S, Tassa A, Qu X, Garuti R, Liang XH, Mizushima N, et al. Bcl-2 antiapoptotic proteins inhibit Beclin 1-dependent autophagy. Cell 2005;122(6) 927-939.

[40] Li Y, Wang Y, Kim E, Beemiller P, Wang CY, Swanson J, et al. Bnip3 mediates the hypoxia-induced inhibition on mammalian target of rapamycin by interacting with Rheb. The Journal of biological chemistry 2007;282(49) 35803-35813.

[41] Sciarretta S, Hariharan N, Monden Y, Zablocki D, Sadoshima J. Is autophagy in response to ischemia and reperfusion protective or detrimental for the heart? Pediatr Cardiol 2011;32(3) 275-281.

[42] Dai W, Hale SL, Kay GL, Jyrala AJ, Kloner RA. Cardioprotective effects of angiotensin II type 1 receptor blockade with olmesartan on reperfusion injury in a rat myocardial ischemia-reperfusion model. Cardiovascular therapeutics 2010;28(1) 30-37.

[43] Yan L, Vatner DE, Kim SJ, Ge H, Masurekar M, Massover WH et al. Autophagy in chronically ischemic myocardium. Proc Natl Acad Sci USA 2005;102(39) 13807-13812.

[44] Scherz-Shouval R, Elazar Z. ROS, mitochondria and the regulation of autophagy. Trends Cell Biol. 2007;17(9) 422-427.

[45] Hamacher-Brady A, Brady NR, Gottlieb RA: Enhancing macroautophagy protects against ischemia/reperfusion injury in cardiac myocytes. J Biol Chem 2006;281(40) 29776-29787.

[46] Javier A. Sala-Mercado, Joseph Wider, Vishnu Vardhan Reddy Undyala, Salik Jahania, Wonsuk Yoo, Robert M. Mentzer, Jr, Roberta A. Gottlieb, and Karin Przyklenk. Profound Cardioprotection with Chloramphenicol Succinate in the Swine Model of Myocardial Ischemia-Reperfusion Injury. Circulation 2010;122(Suppl 11) S179-S184.

[47] Xie Z, Klionsky DJ. Autophagosome formation: core machinery and adaptations. Nat Cell Biol 2007;9(10) 1102-1109.

[48] M, Yamaguchi O, Nakai A, Hikoso S, Takeda T, Mizote I, Oka T, Tamai T, Oyabu J, Murakawa T, Nishida K, Shimizu T, Hori M, Komuro I, Shirasawa T, Mizushima N, Otsu K. Inhibition of autophagy in the heart induces age-related cardiomyopathy. Autophagy 2010;6(5) 600-606.

[49] Dong Y, Undyala VV, Gottlieb RA, Mentzer RM Jr, Przyklenk K. Autophagy: definition, molecular machinery, and potential role in myocardial ischemia-reperfusion injury. J Cardiovasc Pharmacol Ther 2010;15(3) 220-230.

[50] De Meyer GR, De Keulenaer GW, Martinet W. Role of autophagy in heart failure associated with aging. Heart Fail Rev 2010;15(5) 423-430.

[51] Cuervo AM, Bergamini E, Brunk UT, Dröge W, Ffrench M, Terman A. Autophagy and aging: the importance of maintaining "clean" cells. Autophagy 2005;1(3) 131-140.

[52] Gottlieb RA, Finley KD, Mentzer RM Jr. Cardioprotection requires taking out the trash. Basic Res Cardiol 2009;104(2) 169-180.

[53] Gustafsson AB, Gottlieb RA. Autophagy in ischemic heart disease. Circ Res 2009;104(2) 150-158.

[54] Nishida K, Kyoi S, Yamaguchi O, Sadoshima J, Otsu K. The role of autophagy in the heart. Cell Death Differ 2009;16(1) 31-38.

Chapter 10

Progenitor/Stem Cell Engineering for Treatment of Ischemic Heart Diseases: Therapeutic Potentials and Challenges

Yuliang Feng, Yigang Wang and Shi-Zheng Wu

Additional information is available at the end of the chapter

http://dx.doi.org/10.5772/53517

1. Introduction

1.1. Treatment for ischemic heart diseases: State-of-the-art

Cardiovascular diseases, especially ischemic heart disease, are the leading cause of mortality in the United States [1]. In the past decades, pharmacological therapy, such as β-blocker, Angiotensin Converting Enzyme Inhibitor (ACEI)/Angiotensin Receptor Blocker(ARB) have been shown to ameliorate cardiac dysfunction and limit heart remodeling following myocardial infarction [2]. Moreover, the development of coronary artery bypass graft (CABG) can recanalize occlusive coronary and salvage the remaining surviving myocardium [3]. More recently, with the development of percutaneous coronary intervention (PCI), retrograde approach through collaterals has been introduced for percutaneous recanalization of chronic total occlusion (CTO) of the coronary arteries, a new option for the patient with CTO beyond CABG [4]. Unfortunately, even with great advances of these modern technologies, myocardial infarctions will eventually develop into decompensated chronic heart failure. Heart transplantation is currently the last resort for the patient with end-stage heart failure. However, this therapeutic option is limited by donor organ shortage and eventual organ rejection [5]. Therefore, new therapies are required to prevent the progression of pathological remodeling and cell death, as well as to induce tissue recovery in the ischemic heart. Regenerative cardiovascular medicine becomes a holy grail with the goal to replace and repair the damaged myocardium and reverse heart dysfunction. In the past two decades, a variety of stem cells have been investigated by scientists to achieve this goal [6]. Recently developed reprogramming technology, induced pluripotent stem cells (iPSC) has become an alternative source for embryonic stem cells (ESC) without the ethical drawbacks [7], showing their powerful potential to differentiate into desired cell type [8]. A new discipline termed stem cell engineering has recently emerged aiming to reconstruct the damaged heart by integrating progenitor/stem cell biology and bioengineering technology [9]. In this chapter, the recent the recent advances and challenges of progenitor/stem cell engineering for the therapy of ischemic heart disease will be discussed from a translational perspective.

2. Proper cell sources

Appropriate cell sources for stem cell engineering must meet the following requirements: 1) The cell must be electromechanically coupled with the host heart tissue. 2) They must survive in the hostile environment created by ischemic stress [10]. In this regard, several cell types have been tried. Skeletal myoblast was the pioneering attempt but it was found to be limited to contract synchronously with the host myocardium [11]. Bone marrow derived stem cells or hematopoietic stem cells are easily obtained in clinical setting but their potential of cardiogenic differentiation is still being debated [10]. The recent discovery of multipotent cardiac progenitors have been proven to give rise to cardiomyocytes, endothelial, and smooth muscle cells, forming the basic "components" for heart reconstruction [12]. The attempt to discover endogenous cardiac progenitors showed some of those express c-Kit [13, 14] or Sca-1 [14] markers. Transplantation of c-Kit$^+$ cell resulted in neovascularization and cardiomyogenesis in the infarcted heart [13]. Moreover, the cardiosphere obtained from human heart tissue contained a mixed population of c-Kit$^+$ and Sca-1$^+$ cells and could regenerate infarcted heart [15]. These encouraging results led to the initiation of several phase 1 clinical trials: ALCADIA ((AutoLogous Human CArdiac-Derived Stem Cell to Treat Ischemic cArdiomyopathy, NCT00981006), SCIPIO (Cardiac Stem Cell Infusion in Patients with Ischemic Cardiomyopathy) (NCT00474461), and CADUCEUS (NCT00893360). Preliminary data from the SCIPIO and CADUCEUS (CArdiosphere-Derived aUtologous Stem CElls to Reverse ventricUlar dysfunction) trials have been recently published in the *Lancet* [16, 17]. Both studies were aimed to evaluate the feasibility and safety of intracoronary injection of autologous heart-derived cells in a patient post myocardial infarction. The SCIPIO study [16] used c-kit$^+$ cells that were cultured from atrial tissue, whereas the CADUCEUS study [17] is using cardiospheres cultured from biopsy-obtained right ventricular tissue. There is no report related to severe side effect associated with cardiac cell injection in these two studies, although more adverse events were observed in CADUCEUS study (treatment group). Both studies reported reduction in infarct size following cell injection, but only the SCIPIO trial reported an improvement in left ventricular ejection fraction (LVEF). There are still some limitations in these results, as indicated by the limited sample size (16 in SCIPIO and 17 in CADUCEUS) and the absence of a placebo group. Therefore, phase 2 study must be initiated in the future to further confirm its safety and efficacy.

Furthermore, stimulation of the adult progenitor pool with epicardial origin after an acute myocardial infarction (AMI) has been reported with some progress [18-20]. The successful production of iPSC by transducing pluripotent-regulated transcriptional factors has made it a powerful weapon for *ex vivo* expansion of cardiomyocytes [21]. And the direct

http://dx.doi.org/10.5772/53517

differentiation of pluripotent stem cells can be enhanced by administration of BMP4 and activin A [22, 23]. How to remove undifferentiated stem cells from differentiated cardiomyocytes has been a major challenge in translational cardiovascular medicine. Potential solutions to this problem might be can be overcome by i) purification of isl-1^{+} ventricular precursors followed by committed differentiation [24] or ii) transgenic enrichment via negative selection of iPSC using a suicide gene (thymidine kinase)/positive selection of cardiomyocytes expressing a bicistronic reporter GFP expression under control of alpha myosin heavy chain promoter [25]. Taken together, these cells provide a valuable source for generation of a cell sheet/patch for tissue engineering purpose. Therefore, there are two techniques commonly used for cardiac repair. The first is transplantation of stem cells with cardiogenic potential into injured heart or pre-induction of stem cells into cardiomyocytes followed by implantation. The second is stimulation of the endogenous cardiac progenitor pool to propagate cardiovascular offspring. More recently, the laboratories of Deepak Srivastava and Eric Olson reported a new method, termed by "in vivo reprogramming of cardiomyocytes", making *in vivo* transformation of scar tissue into beating heart muscle possible. By transducing with retroviruses encoding GMT (GATA4, MEF2C, TBX5) [26] or GMTH (GMT+Hand2) [27] *in vivo* following left anterior descending artery (LAD) ligation, cardiac fibroblasts, the natural "partner" of cardiomyocytes, become activated, migrate to the injured site, and proliferate, thus rendering these cells susceptible to retroviral infection and subsequent epigenetic reprogramming event. Both groups reported a significant conversion of transduced fibroblasts, identified by genetic lineage tracing of non-cardiomyocyte in the heart, to an "induced cardiomyocyte-like (iCM)" or "induced cardiac-like myocyte (iCLM)" state iCMs/iCLMs. Although without presence of rhythm disorder in mice, it is necessary to test the approach in pigs, whose hearts are similar to those of human in terms of size and physiology, to further evaluate its efficacy and safety before clinical trial.

3. Engineering approach

Direct injection of cell suspension into infarcted area or peri-infarcted area is still the main progenitor/stem cell treatment used for cardiac repair. Nevertheless, the poor survival of stem cells in the harsh environment (hypoxia, inflammatory cytokines, etc.) limits the reparative function of progenitor/stem cells in ischemic heart [28].

Combining progenitor/stem cell biology and bioengineering, tissue engineering holds great promise to generate viable three dimensional heart tissue with vasculature prior to engraftment to the heart, as an integral part of the host. This tissue graft should display contractile and electromechanical coupled properties, contributing to the improvement of heart function. The recent evidence from large animals indicated that human ES-derived cardiomyocytes electrically coupled and suppressed arrhythmias in injured hearts. This provided support for the continued development of human stem cell derived tissue graft for cardiac repair [29]. The conventional approach involved seeding cell on scaffolds and culture *in vitro* prior to implantation.

Eschenhagen and Zimmermann constructed an engineering heart tissue (EHT) by seeding neonatal rat cardiomyocytes and a mix of collagen I, extracellular matrix proteins (Matrigel) into a lattices or circular molds. Upon spontaneous remodeling of the liquid reconstitution mixture and cyclic mechanical, EHT spontaneously and synchronously contracted after one to two weeks of cultivation, which highlights the great importance of physical stimulation on the maintenance of the physical and mechanical function of EHT [30]. This pioneering work for the first time showed EHT could ameliorate cardiac function post MI.

3.1. Scaffold free tissue construct

The use of cell sheets provides a simple scaffold-free approach by seeding cardiac cells on poly (N-isopropylacrylamide)-grafted polystyrene dishes and then lowering the temperature to 20ºC, thus inducing the detachment of intact cell monolayers without enzymatic digestion. Using this method, a 1-mm-thick cell patch can be created by serial stacking of multiple monolayer sheets [31]. A recent study by Murry group using ESC-derived cardiomyocytes reported another scaffold free approach, demonstrating cell aggregation is sufficient to generate functional EHT also showing endothelial cell and fibroblast are required for the survival and integration of EHT and in host myocardium [32]. Further studies are needed to optimize the proportion of cardiomyocyte, endothelial cells, and fibroblast for maximal performance of EHT.

3.2. Construction of myocardial tissue/heart using decellularized native tissue

In order to create decellularized scaffolds, Taylor and her team perfused rat hearts with detergents to remove the cells and leave a complex architecture of acellular extracellular matrix (ECM) behind. [33]. This native scaffold was reseeded with cardiomyocytes and endothelial cells taken from rats. They then placed these constructs in bioreactors that simulated blood pressure, electrical stimulation, and other aspects of cardiac physiology to assure integration of the scaffold and seeded cells. Although approximately only 2% of normal contractile activity was acquired from this approach, this is a successful proof-of-concept trial and might be the ultimate biomimetic method for constructing an intact human heart.

3.3. Porous scaffolds

By using electrical stimulation, Vunjak-Novakovic *et al.*, established a method to assemble individual cardiomyocytes into a functional cell patch [34]. The hydrogel-encapsulated neonatal rat heart cells were cultivated on porous collagen scaffolds. Currently, this methodology has been applied in other cell types (e.g. hESC) [35] and with other scaffold material (e.g. synthetic elastomers) [36]. 3 days before electrical stimulation, the cells were cultured in petri dishes to allow sufficient expression of gap junction protein (e.g. Cx43) and other molecules involved in contraction. Then the cells were subjected to electrical stimulation to induce synchronous contraction and alteration of structural organization, resulting in the formation of mature myocardium with elongated, viable cells aligned in parallel.

3.4. Biological and synthetic polymers

Collagen is the first biological polymer used for fabrication of three dimensional tissues. It was reported that neonatal rat cardiomyocytes spontaneously contracted when cultivated in gelatin coated scaffold. Although the implanted cardiomyocytes survived in infarcted heart, LVEF is not significantly improved after long term observation. Furthermore, Zimmermann's group engineered contractile 3-D heart tissue, in which cardiomyocytes encapsulated with ring--shaped hydrogels (collagen and Matrigel) showing reduction of ventricle dilatation, significant ventricular wall thickening and improvement of the fractional shortening (FS) [30]. The improvement of cardiac function, myofibril organization indicated that mechanical stimulation is important for maturation of myocardial structure. Leor et al. also reported that 3-D alginate scaffolds seeded with fetal rat cardiomyocytes attenuated left ventricular dilatation and deterioration of the heart function after myocardial infarction [37].

4. Progenitor/stem cell niche engineering

As we discussed above, the laboratories of Deepak Srivastava and Eric Olson were successful in reprogramming cardiac fibroblasts *in vivo* into cardiomyocytes with a significant efficiency. In 2010, Deepak's team attempted to reprogram cardiac fibroblast into cardiomyocytes with the same combination of transcription factors *in vitro* but experienced low efficiency [38], while recently Sean M. Wu's team reported in some cases, the reprogramming is still inefficiency [39]. The great difference with respect to reprogramming efficiency *in vitro* and *in vivo* using the same transcription factor cocktail suggested that the local microenvironment (niche) is a critical checkpoint for cell reprogramming and regeneration. *In vivo*, the stem cell niche is a complex and dynamic unit, and how these components interact to modulate progenitor/stem cell fate is on the horizon to be understood. Alteration of the properties of progenitor/stem cell niches may provide new therapeutic strategies for progenitor/stem cell engineering by interrupting cardiac remodeling or accelerating the reparative process. Here we discuss two key expects of progenitor/stem cell niche, namely mechanical cue and chemical cues and their implication for progenitor/stem cell engineering.

4.1. Matrix rigidity

Progenitor/stem cell engineering involves coordination of selective proliferation of precursor/stem cells and differentiation into target somatic cells (cardiomyocytes, smooth muscle cell, and endothelial cells). Mechanical cues influence proliferation, differentiation, migration, and spatial morphological organization. These cues include the rigidity of the surrounding matrix or cell adhesion substratum. Thus, better understanding of the role of matrix rigidity is critical for optimization of the regimes of mechanical conditioning of cultured tissue constructs. Based on a pioneering study which discovered mechanosensitive transcriptional mechanism in 2009 [40], Kshitiz *et al* showed that resident cardiac progenitor cells continually monitored cell substratum rigidity and demonstrated enhanced proliferation, endothelial differentiation, and morphogenesis when the cell substratum rigidity closely matched that of myocardium [41].

This process is mediated by p190RhoGAP, a guanosine triphosphatase–activating protein for RhoA, acting through RhoA-dependent and -independent mechanisms. Downregulation of p190RhoGAP triggered a series of developmental events by coupling cell-cell and cell-substratum interactions to genetic circuits controlling differentiation. Hence, preconditioning of endothelial progenitors could change p190RhoGAP abundance and thus promote angiogenesis in engrafted heart. More generally, the results suggest the importance of the feedback between the rigidity of a developing or regenerating tissue and the control of cell growth and differentiation, which may be critical for adaptive development and maintenance of structurally complex tissues and organs.

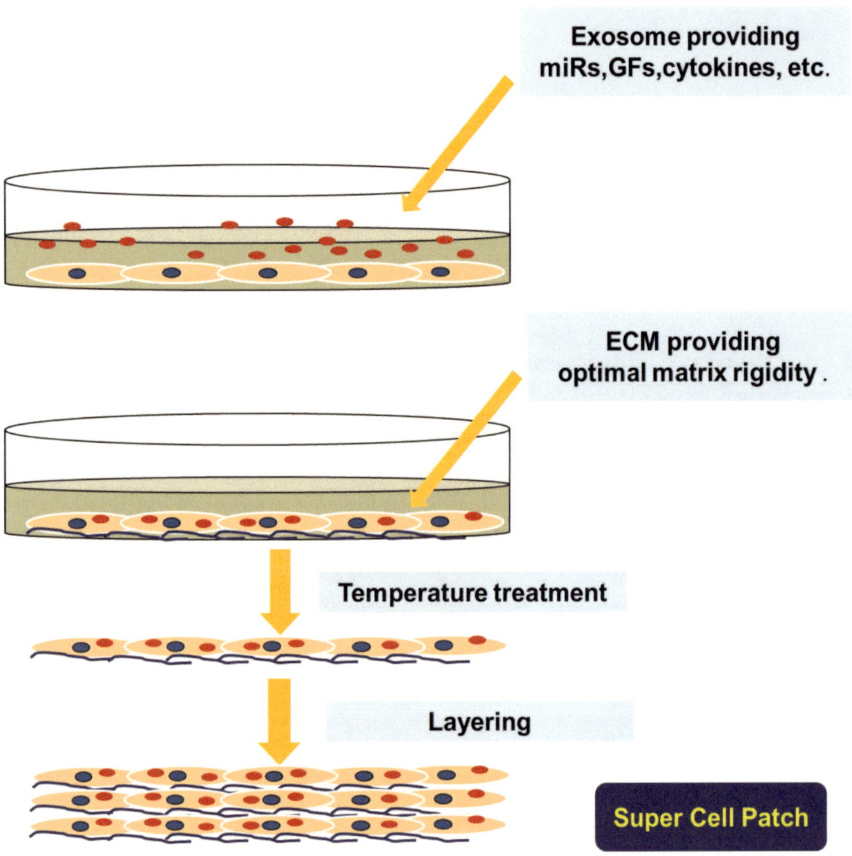

Figure 1. Fabrication of "Super Cell Patch". Progenitor/cells were treated with exosome containing microRNAs (miRs), growth factors (GFs) and cytokines etc. Then the progenitor/stem cells were administered with optimized ECM to provide the suitable matrix rigidity for engraftment. Subsequently, confluent cells forming sheets were released from the dish surface by decreasing temperature from 37ºC to 20ºC. Then, several cell sheets were stratified and placed across the epicardial surface of infarcted myocardium to form a functional bridge for the purpose of restoring global contractile function.

http://dx.doi.org/10.5772/53517

4.2. Exosome secretion

Recent studies have suggested four potential mechanisms for how exogenous-culture-expanded MSC may contribute to cardiovascular repair: transdifferentiation, cell fusion with a native cell, stimulation of endogenous cardiac progenitor/stem cells via direct cell-cell communication or paracrine mechanism [42]. Transdifferentiation of MSC into cardiomyocytes is not inefficient in current regimes [10]. Cell fusion is a rare event[43]. As aforementioned, the observed salutary effects of progenitor/stem cell on cardiac repair probably resulted from paracrine mechanism. And the cardiogenic differentiation of CSC stimulated by MSC processed a limited capacity [44]. By antibody array and Liquid Chromatography with Tandem Mass Spectrometry Detection (LC-MS/MS), compelling evidences have shown MSC could secrete a wide spectrum of trophic proteins that could induce proliferation and differentiation of CPC and angiogenesis [45]. Interestingly, in 2007, the paper published on *Nature Cell Biology* revealed mRNAs and microRNAs in the exosome (the major microvesicle for intercellular communication) can be delivered from one cell to another, and can be functional in this new location [46]. This hallmark study elicited amazing expansion of studies on exosomes in the last 3 years, making it a very exciting field now. A recent study has targeted exosomes to the brain to treat Alzheimer's disease by engineering exosomes with dendrite cells marker [47]. This study highlighted the possibility that cardiac-specific exosomes can be engineered to treat ischemic heart diseases without any risk of immunorejection or carcinogenesis by viral infection. Thus, compared to the delivery of single growth factors or cytokines, the direct administration of exosomes derived from preconditioned progenitors/stem cells into ischemic heart or using cell sheet/patch modified with preconditioned exosomes might be a new trend to improve cardiac repair in a more efficient way (Fig. 1).

5. Conclusions

Progenitor/stem cell engineering has presented as an exciting and promising avenue for the treatment of ischemic heart diseases. Regeneration of damaged heart by progenitor/stem cell engineering is becoming a fact rather than fiction. The translation of experimental discovery in progenitor/stem cell engineering into clinical application should be accelerated and large scale clinical trials should be initiated in the patients with ischemic heart diseases. Therefore, the collaboration of progenitor/stem cell biologists, bioengineers, and physicians is possibly the future modality in personalized regenerative medicine.

Acknowledgements

Funding sources

This work was supported by NIH grants, HL089824, HL081859, HL110740 (Y. Wang).

Mianna Armstrong for technical assistance.

Author details

Yuliang Feng[1,2], Yigang Wang[1*] and Shi-Zheng Wu[3]

*Address all correspondence to: yi-gang.wang @uc.edu

1 Department of Pathology and Laboratory Medicine, College of Medicine, University of Cincinnati, Cincinnati, Ohio, USA

2 Medical Research Center of Guangdong General Hospital, Guangdong Academy of Medical Sciences, Guangdong Provincial Cardiovascular Institute, Southern Medical University, Guangzhou, China

3 Qinghai Provincial People's Hospital, Qinghai Clinical Medical Institute, Xining, Qinghai, China

References

[1] Roger, V. L, Go, A. S, Lloyd-jones, D. M, Adams, R. J, Berry, J. D, Brown, T. M, et al. Heart disease and stroke statistics--2011 update: a report from the American Heart Association. Circulation. (Journal Article). (2011). e, 18-209.

[2] Adding ACEIs and/or ARBs to Standard Therapy for Stable Ischemic Heart Disease: Benefits and HarmsBook Chapter). (2007).

[3] Mcmurray, J. J. Heart failure in 2011: Heart failure therapy--technology to the fore. Nat Rev Cardiol. (Journal Article; Review). (2012)., 9(2), 73-4.

[4] Jones, D. A, Weerackody, R, Rathod, K, Behar, J, Gallagher, S, Knight, C. J, et al. Successful recanalization of chronic total occlusions is associated with improved long-term survival. JACC Cardiovasc Interv. (Journal Article). (2012)., 5(4), 380-8.

[5] Jessup, M, Albert, N. M, Lanfear, D. E, Lindenfeld, J, Massie, B. M, Walsh, M. N, et al. ACCF/AHA/HFSA 2011 survey results: current staffing profile of heart failure programs, including programs that perform heart transplant and mechanical circulatory support device implantation. J Card Fail. (Comparative Study; Journal Article; Multicenter Study). (2011)., 17(5), 349-58.

[6] Ptaszek, L. M, Mansour, M, Ruskin, J. N, & Chien, K. R. Towards regenerative therapy for cardiac disease. Lancet. (Journal Article; Research Support, Non-U.S. Gov't; Review). (2012)., 379(9819), 933-42.

[7] Takahashi, K, Tanabe, K, Ohnuki, M, Narita, M, Ichisaka, T, Tomoda, K, et al. Induction of pluripotent stem cells from adult human fibroblasts by defined factors. Cell. (Journal Article; Research Support, Non-U.S. Gov't). (2007)., 131(5), 861-72.

[8] Bilic, J, & Izpisua, B. J. Concise review: Induced pluripotent stem cells versus embryonic stem cells: close enough or yet too far apart? Stem Cells. (Journal Article; Research Support, Non-U.S. Gov't; Review). (2012). , 30(1), 33-41.

[9] Sui, R, Liao, X, Zhou, X, & Tan, Q. The current status of engineering myocardial tissue. Stem Cell Rev. (Journal Article; Review). (2011). , 7(1), 172-80.

[10] Laflamme, M. A, & Murry, C. E. Heart regeneration. Nature. (Journal Article; Research Support, N.I.H., Extramural; Review). (2011). , 473(7347), 326-35.

[11] Formigli, L, Zecchi-orlandini, S, Meacci, E, & Bani, D. Skeletal myoblasts for heart regeneration and repair: state of the art and perspectives on the mechanisms for functional cardiac benefits. Curr Pharm Des. (Journal Article; Review). (2010). , 16(8), 915-28.

[12] Hansson, E. M, Lindsay, M. E, & Chien, K. R. Regeneration next: toward heart stem cell therapeutics. Cell Stem Cell. (Journal Article; Research Support, N.I.H., Extramural; Research Support, Non-U.S. Gov't; Review). (2009). , 5(4), 364-77.

[13] Beltrami, A. P, Barlucchi, L, Torella, D, Baker, M, Limana, F, Chimenti, S, et al. Adult cardiac stem cells are multipotent and support myocardial regeneration. Cell. (Journal Article; Research Support, U.S. Gov't, P.H.S.). (2003). , 114(6), 763-76.

[14] Oh, H, Bradfute, S. B, Gallardo, T. D, Nakamura, T, Gaussin, V, Mishina, Y, et al. Cardiac progenitor cells from adult myocardium: homing, differentiation, and fusion after infarction. Proc Natl Acad Sci U S A. (In Vitro; Journal Article; Research Support, Non-U.S. Gov't; Research Support, U.S. Gov't, P.H.S.). (2003). , 100(21), 12313-8.

[15] Chimenti, I, Smith, R. R, Li, T. S, Gerstenblith, G, Messina, E, Giacomello, A, et al. Relative roles of direct regeneration versus paracrine effects of human cardiosphere-derived cells transplanted into infarcted mice. Circ Res. (Journal Article; Research Support, N.I.H., Extramural; Research Support, Non-U.S. Gov't). (2010). , 106(5), 971-80.

[16] Bolli, R, Chugh, A. R, Amario, D, Loughran, D, Stoddard, J. H, & Ikram, M. F. S, et al. Cardiac stem cells in patients with ischaemic cardiomyopathy (SCIPIO): initial results of a randomised phase 1 trial. Lancet. (Clinical Trial, Phase I; Journal Article; Randomized Controlled Trial; Research Support, N.I.H., Extramural; Research Support, Non-U.S. Gov't). (2011). , 378(9806), 1847-57.

[17] Makkar, R. R, Smith, R. R, Cheng, K, Malliaras, K, Thomson, L. E, Berman, D, et al. Intracoronary cardiosphere-derived cells for heart regeneration after myocardial infarction (CADUCEUS): a prospective, randomised phase 1 trial. Lancet. (Clinical Trial, Phase I; Journal Article; Multicenter Study; Randomized Controlled Trial; Research Support, N.I.H., Extramural; Research Support, Non-U.S. Gov't). (2012). , 379(9819), 895-904.

[18] Zhou, B, Ma, Q, Rajagopal, S, Wu, S. M, Domian, I, Rivera-feliciano, J, et al. Epicardial progenitors contribute to the cardiomyocyte lineage in the developing heart. Na-

ture. (Journal Article; Research Support, N.I.H., Extramural; Research Support, Non-U.S. Gov't). (2008)., 454(7200), 109-13.

[19] Smart, N, Bollini, S, Dube, K. N, Vieira, J. M, Zhou, B, Davidson, S, et al. De novo cardiomyocytes from within the activated adult heart after injury. Nature. (Journal Article; Research Support, Non-U.S. Gov't). (2011)., 474(7353), 640-4.

[20] Zhou, B, Honor, L. B, He, H, Ma, Q, Oh, J. H, Butterfield, C, et al. Adult mouse epicardium modulates myocardial injury by secreting paracrine factors. J Clin Invest. (Journal Article; Research Support, N.I.H., Extramural; Research Support, Non-U.S. Gov't). (2011)., 121(5), 1894-904.

[21] Burridge, P. W, Keller, G, Gold, J. D, & Wu, J. C. Production of de novo cardiomyocytes: human pluripotent stem cell differentiation and direct reprogramming. Cell Stem Cell. (Journal Article; Research Support, N.I.H., Extramural; Research Support, Non-U.S. Gov't). (2012)., 10(1), 16-28.

[22] Yang, L, Soonpaa, M. H, Adler, E. D, Roepke, T. K, Kattman, S. J, Kennedy, M, et al. Human cardiovascular progenitor cells develop from a KDR+ embryonic-stem-cell-derived population. Nature. (Journal Article; Research Support, N.I.H., Extramural). (2008)., 453(7194), 524-8.

[23] Laflamme, M. A, Chen, K. Y, Naumova, A. V, Muskheli, V, Fugate, J. A, Dupras, S. K, et al. Cardiomyocytes derived from human embryonic stem cells in pro-survival factors enhance function of infarcted rat hearts. Nat Biotechnol. (Journal Article; Research Support, N.I.H., Extramural; Research Support, Non-U.S. Gov't). (2007). , 25(9), 1015-24.

[24] Moretti, A, Bellin, M, Jung, C. B, Thies, T. M, Takashima, Y, Bernshausen, A, et al. Mouse and human induced pluripotent stem cells as a source for multipotent Isl1+ cardiovascular progenitors. Faseb J. (Journal Article; Research Support, Non-U.S. Gov't). (2010)., 24(3), 700-11.

[25] Cheng, F, Ke, Q, Chen, F, Cai, B, Gao, Y, Ye, C, et al. Protecting against wayward human induced pluripotent stem cells with a suicide gene. Biomaterials. (Journal Article; Research Support, Non-U.S. Gov't). (2012)., 33(11), 3195-204.

[26] Qian, L, Huang, Y, Spencer, C. I, Foley, A, Vedantham, V, Liu, L, et al. In vivo reprogramming of murine cardiac fibroblasts into induced cardiomyocytes. Nature. (Journal Article; Research Support, N.I.H., Extramural; Research Support, Non-U.S. Gov't). (2012)., 485(7400), 593-8.

[27] Song, K, Nam, Y. J, Luo, X, Qi, X, Tan, W, Huang, G. N, et al. Heart repair by reprogramming non-myocytes with cardiac transcription factors. Nature. (Journal Article; Research Support, N.I.H., Extramural; Research Support, Non-U.S. Gov't). (2012). , 485(7400), 599-604.

[28] Choi, S. H, Jung, S. Y, Kwon, S. M, & Baek, S. H. Perspectives on stem cell therapy for cardiac regeneration. Advances and challenges. Circ J. (Journal Article; Research Support, Non-U.S. Gov't). (2012)., 76(6), 1307-12.

[29] Shiba, Y, Fernandes, S, Zhu, W. Z, Filice, D, Muskheli, V, Kim, J, et al. Human ES-cell-derived cardiomyocytes electrically couple and suppress arrhythmias in injured hearts. Nature. (JOURNAL ARTICLE). (2012).

[30] Zimmermann, W. H, Schneiderbanger, K, Schubert, P, Didie, M, Munzel, F, Heubach, J. F, et al. Tissue engineering of a differentiated cardiac muscle construct. Circ Res. (Journal Article; Research Support, Non-U.S. Gov't). (2002)., 90(2), 223-30.

[31] Haraguchi, Y, Shimizu, T, Sasagawa, T, Sekine, H, Sakaguchi, K, Kikuchi, T, et al. Fabrication of functional three-dimensional tissues by stacking cell sheets in vitro. Nat Protoc. (Journal Article; Research Support, Non-U.S. Gov't). (2012)., 7(5), 850-8.

[32] Stevens, K. R, Pabon, L, Muskheli, V, & Murry, C. E. Scaffold-free human cardiac tissue patch created from embryonic stem cells. Tissue Eng Part A. (Journal Article; Research Support, N.I.H., Extramural; Research Support, Non-U.S. Gov't). (2009). , 15(6), 1211-22.

[33] Ott, H. C, Matthiesen, T. S, Goh, S. K, Black, L. D, Kren, S. M, Netoff, T. I, et al. Perfusion-decellularized matrix: using nature's platform to engineer a bioartificial heart. Nat Med. (Journal Article; Research Support, Non-U.S. Gov't). (2008)., 14(2), 213-21.

[34] Radisic, M, Park, H, Shing, H, Consi, T, Schoen, F. J, Langer, R, et al. Functional assembly of engineered myocardium by electrical stimulation of cardiac myocytes cultured on scaffolds. Proc Natl Acad Sci U S A. (Journal Article; Research Support, Non-U.S. Gov't; Research Support, U.S. Gov't, Non-P.H.S.; Research Support, U.S. Gov't, P.H.S.). (2004)., 101(52), 18129-34.

[35] Serena, E, Figallo, E, Tandon, N, Cannizzaro, C, Gerecht, S, Elvassore, N, et al. Electrical stimulation of human embryonic stem cells: cardiac differentiation and the generation of reactive oxygen species. Exp Cell Res. (Journal Article; Research Support, N.I.H., Extramural; Research Support, Non-U.S. Gov't). (2009)., 315(20), 3611-9.

[36] Tandon, N, Cannizzaro, C, Chao, P. H, Maidhof, R, Marsano, A, Au, H. T, et al. Electrical stimulation systems for cardiac tissue engineering. Nat Protoc. (Journal Article; Research Support, N.I.H., Extramural; Research Support, Non-U.S. Gov't). (2009). , 4(2), 155-73.

[37] Leor, J, Tuvia, S, Guetta, V, Manczur, F, Castel, D, Willenz, U, et al. Intracoronary injection of in situ forming alginate hydrogel reverses left ventricular remodeling after myocardial infarction in Swine. J Am Coll Cardiol. (Journal Article; Research Support, Non-U.S. Gov't). (2009)., 54(11), 1014-23.

[38] Ieda, M, Fu, J. D, Delgado-olguin, P, Vedantham, V, Hayashi, Y, Bruneau, B. G, et al. Direct reprogramming of fibroblasts into functional cardiomyocytes by defined fac-

tors. Cell. (Journal Article; Research Support, N.I.H., Extramural; Research Support, Non-U.S. Gov't). (2010)., 142(3), 375-86.

[39] Chen, J. X, Krane, M, Deutsch, M. A, Wang, L, Rav-acha, M, Gregoire, S, et al. Inefficient reprogramming of fibroblasts into cardiomyocytes using Gata4, Mef2c, and Tbx5. Circ Res. (Journal Article; Research Support, N.I.H., Extramural; Research Support, Non-U.S. Gov't). (2012)., 111(1), 50-5.

[40] Mammoto, A, Connor, K. M, Mammoto, T, Yung, C. W, Huh, D, Aderman, C. M, et al. A mechanosensitive transcriptional mechanism that controls angiogenesis. Nature. (Journal Article; Research Support, N.I.H., Extramural; Research Support, Non-U.S. Gov't; Research Support, U.S. Gov't, Non-P.H.S.). (2009)., 457(7233), 1103-8.

[41] KshitizHubbi ME, Ahn EH, Downey J, Afzal J, Kim DH, et al. Matrix rigidity controls endothelial differentiation and morphogenesis of cardiac precursors. Sci Signal. (Journal Article; Research Support, N.I.H., Extramural; Research Support, Non-U.S. Gov't). (2012). a41.

[42] Gnecchi, M, Danieli, P, & Cervio, E. Mesenchymal stem cell therapy for heart disease. Vascul Pharmacol. (Journal Article; Research Support, Non-U.S. Gov't). (2012). , 57(1), 48-55.

[43] Noiseux, N, Gnecchi, M, Lopez-ilasaca, M, Zhang, L, Solomon, S. D, Deb, A, et al. Mesenchymal stem cells overexpressing Akt dramatically repair infarcted myocardium and improve cardiac function despite infrequent cellular fusion or differentiation. Mol Ther. (Journal Article; Research Support, N.I.H., Extramural; Research Support, Non-U.S. Gov't). (2006)., 14(6), 840-50.

[44] Mazhari, R, & Hare, J. M. Mechanisms of action of mesenchymal stem cells in cardiac repair: potential influences on the cardiac stem cell niche. Nat Clin Pract Cardiovasc Med. (Journal Article; Research Support, N.I.H., Extramural; Research Support, Non-U.S. Gov't). (2007). Suppl 1:S, 21-6.

[45] Lee, M. J, Kim, J, Kim, M. Y, Bae, Y. S, Ryu, S. H, Lee, T. G, et al. Proteomic analysis of tumor necrosis factor-alpha-induced secretome of human adipose tissue-derived mesenchymal stem cells. J Proteome Res. (Journal Article; Research Support, Non-U.S. Gov't). (2010)., 9(4), 1754-62.

[46] Valadi, H, Ekstrom, K, Bossios, A, Sjostrand, M, Lee, J. J, & Lotvall, J. O. Exosome-mediated transfer of mRNAs and microRNAs is a novel mechanism of genetic exchange between cells. Nat Cell Biol. (Journal Article; Research Support, Non-U.S. Gov't). (2007)., 9(6), 654-9.

[47] Alvarez-erviti, L, Seow, Y, Yin, H, Betts, C, Lakhal, S, & Wood, M. J. Delivery of siRNA to the mouse brain by systemic injection of targeted exosomes. Nat Biotechnol. (Journal Article; Research Support, Non-U.S. Gov't). (2011)., 29(4), 341-5.

Chapter 11

Role of Fatty Acid Imaging with ^{123}I- β-methyl-p-^{123}I-Iodophenyl-Pentadecanoic Acid (^{123}I-BMIPP) in Ischemic Heart Diseases

Junichi Taki, Ichiro Matsunari, Hiroshi Wakabayashi,
Anri Inaki and Seigo Kinuya

Additional information is available at the end of the chapter

http://dx.doi.org/10.5772/53548

1. Introduction

In nuclear cardiology, myocardial perfusion imaging has been widely and thoroughly investigated and used in various heart diseases, especially in ischemic heart diseases. However, beyond perfusion imaging, myocardial fatty acid metabolic imaging may yield valuable insight into the pathologic process of various heart diseases including ischemic heart diseases, cardiomyopathy, and diabetic heart etc [1, 2].

To run the contractile machinery and ion pumps to maintain rhythmic beating and integrity of the myocardium, the healthy heart derives its energy from a variety of oxidizable substrates such as fatty acids, glucose, lactate, amino acids etc. Approximately two-thirds or more of the total energy produced by myocardium is derived from fatty acid oxidation and the most of the remaining energy is covered by the glucose metabolism. Both fatty acid and glucose are catabolized to acetyl-COA through beta-oxidation and glycolysis and the metabolite is oxidized in the tricarboxylic acid (TCA) cycle (Fig 1). To respond the constantly changing environmental conditions and energy demands, the heart maintains the balance between its energetic supply and demands by shifting fluxes through existing various metabolic pathways. Short-term modulation of substrate switching is based on an effective interplay between various substrates, with metabolism of one substrate automatically suppressing the pathway of another substrate via rapid enzymatic changes. In the postprandial and under resting conditions, long-chain fatty acids are the predominant energy substrate for adult heart. On the other hand, during exercise or stress, predominant energy source shifts to carbohydrate [3] because the efficiency of glucose as substrate exceeds the efficiency of fatty acids as substrate by as much as 40% [4]. In ischemia, oxidative metabolism of free fatty acid is decreased because β-oxidation of fatty acid in mitochondria requires a large amount of oxygen, and glucose becomes the preferred substrate for anaerobic glycolysis that requires less oxygen consumption [5,6]. This metabolic switch from predominat fatty acid use to predominant glucose use seems crucial in preserving myocardial viability. (Fig 2) Therefore, different imaging tracers that permit direct assessment of myocardial metabolism are desired to evaluate the pathophysiological changes in various heart disease. Current available tracers for metabolic imaging are several fatty acid tracers, ^{18}F-FDG for the evaluation of glucose metabolism, and ^{11}C-acetate for the assessment of oxygen consumption. Of these tracers, only ^{123}I-labeled fatty acid tracers are currently available for SPECT imaging. In this chapter, basic characteristics and clinical value of ^{123}I-labeld fatty acid agents, especially β-methyl-p-^{123}I-iodophenyl-pentadecanoic acid (BMIPP) follows.

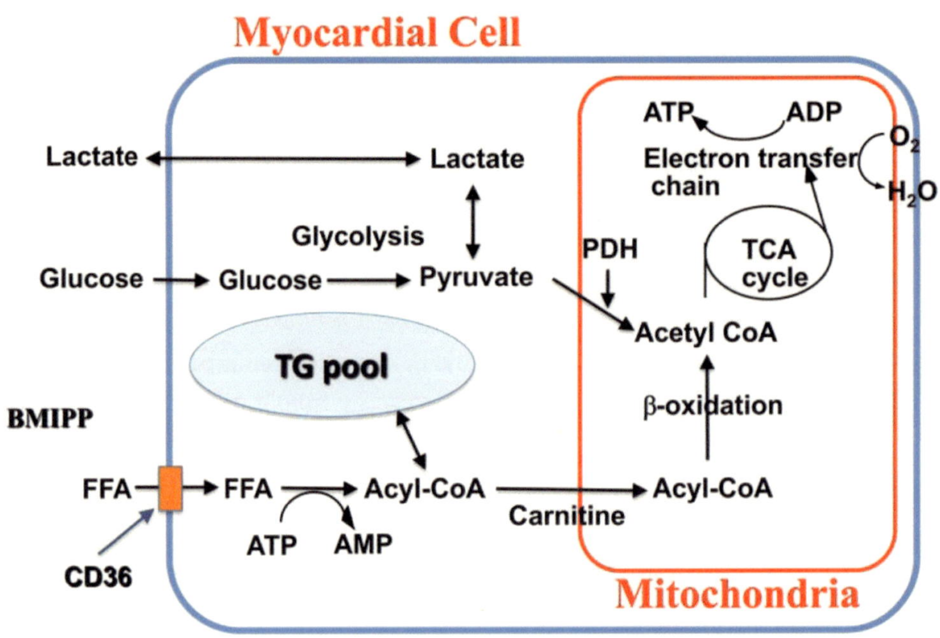

Figure 1. Schematic presentation of substrates metabolism in myocardium. ADP = adenosine diphosphate, AMP = adenosine monophosphate, ATP = adenosine triphosphate, BMIPP = β-methyl-iodophenyl-pentadecanoic acid, CoA = coenzyme A, FFA = free fatty acid, PDH = pyruvate dehydrogenase, TCA = tricarboxylic acid, TG = triglyceride

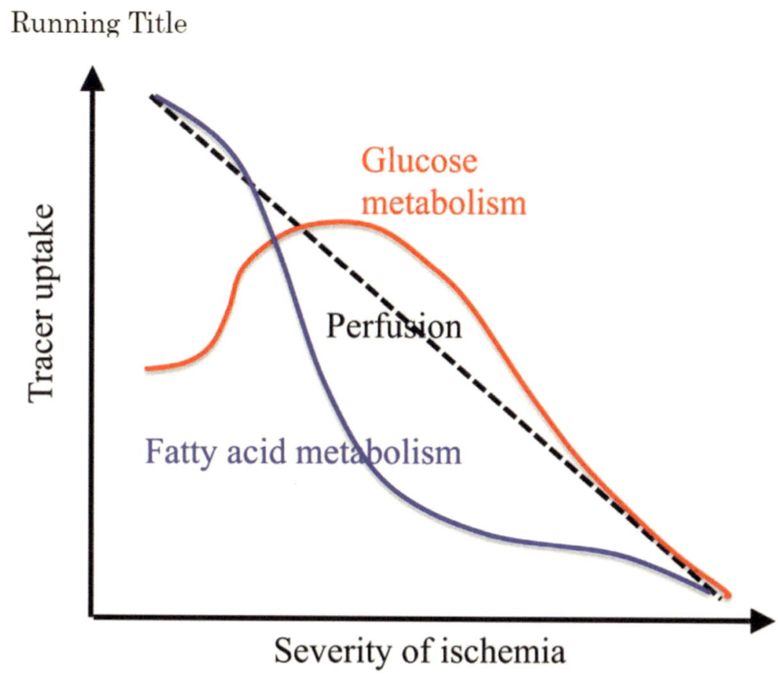

Figure 2. Relation between myocardial perfusion and fatty acid and glucose metabolism.

When myocardial perfusion decreases, fatty acid metabolism can not be maintained because β-oxidation of fatty acid in mitochondria requires a large amount of oxygen, and glucose becomes the preferred substrate for anaerobic glycolysis that requires less oxygen consumption. Therefore, the decrease in tracer uptake for fatty acid substrate analogue such as BMIPP becomes more prominent than the decrease of perfusion tracer. On the contrary, anaerobic glucose metabolism relatively increases, presenting increased or preserved FDG uptake in the area with reduced perfusion. When myocardial perfusion decreases further, glucose anaerobic metabolism also declines finally and myocardial viability will be lost eventually.

2. Myocardial fatty acid metabolism

Although the primary sources of energy are lactate and glucose for fetal heart, fatty acids comprise 60% to 80% of the energy source in adult heart to run the contractile machinery and ion pumps to maintain rhythmic beating and integrity of the myocardium [7].

Due to hydrophobic nature of fatty acids, they are delivered to the heart by binding to plasma albumin or lipoproteins. After dissociating from albumin or lipoprotein, fatty acids can pass through the sarcolemmal membrane by diffusion or a facilitated transport mechanism. The fatty acid translocase CD36 was suggested that it accounts for the key uptake mechanism of long-chain fatty acid through the analysis of minority of patients with absent uptake of ^{123}I-BMIPP (15-(p-iodophenyl)-3(R, S)-methylpentadecanoic acid) even without significant cardiac abnormality [8,9] The patients with deficient myocardial uptake of BMIPP has been proved to correspond to the patients with type I CD36 deficiency (neither platelets nor monocytes expresse CD36) [10-12] and biopsy specimen from the patients with absent myocardial BMIPP uptake and type I CD36 deficiency demonstrated no expression of CD36 on the myocardial capillary endothelial cells [13]. These patients without BMIPP cardiac uptake showed compensatory increased FDG uptake [14,15] and several gene abnormalities related to CD36 deficiency have been reported [16,17]. Based on these clinical data and other animal experiments, it has been proved that CD36 plays a crucial role in fatty acid transport into the cells [18].

Once the fatty acid is taken up by the myocyte, it undergoes adenosine triphosphate (ATP) dependent conversion to acyl-CoAs and are consequently trapped inside the cell. Then the acyl-CoAs are taken up by mithochondria via an acyl carnitine carrier system and is rapidly catabolized by β-oxidation into 2-carbon fragments, acetyl-CoAs, which enter the TCA cycle for further oxidation to become water and carbon dioxide. (Fig 1) The half-life of β-oxidation is fast and in the order of minutes, but is dependent on the adequate oxygen availability. The remainder of the total fatty acid entering the myocyte is incorporated into the lipid pool, mainly in the form of triglycerides and phospholipids, or into myocardial structural lipids and presents in the myocardium for a long time. Turnover in the lipid pool is much slower with the half-life of the order of hours.

3. Tracers for fatty acid imaging for SPECT (Fig 3)

In mid 1970's, several iodinated long chain fatty acids were developed by introducing radioiodine to the terminal position of fatty acids without altering extraction efficiency compared with the natural compound [19-21]. These straight chain fatty acids, ^{123}I-hexadecanoic acid (IHXA) and ^{123}I -heptadecanoic acid (IHDA) were proved to be an indicator of myocardial perfusion in canine model and human [20,21]. After rapid initial myocardial extraction these traces showed biexponential clearance similar to that of ^{11}C-palmitate with rapid and slow components, those were thought to represent β-oxidation of fatty acids and fatty acids storage in lipid pool, respectively. However, a canine study suggested that washout rate of radioactivity from the heart reflected the back diffusion of deiodinated free iodine not by β-oxidation [20]. A clinical study with IHDA demonstrated high image quality early after injection but it deteriorated rapidly because of rapid reduction of myocardial counts and increase in background counts by deiodinated radioiodine [23]. Accordingly, these characteristics of the tracers make IHDA and IHXA unattractive for clinical use, especially for SPECT study.

To overcome the problem of these alkyl fatty acids, the phenyl fatty acid was developed by attaching iodide to the para position of phenyl ring (IPPA) [24]. Because this agent demonstrates high myocardial uptake without essential release of free radioiodide into circulation, the image quality is excellent. Animal experiment demonstrated that the IPPA accumulated rapidly to myocardium followed by a two-component tracer clearance similar to ^{14}C-palmitate, permitting estimation of metabolic rate [25]. The uptake of IPPA during exercise is related to myocardial perfusion and its catabolism follows the usual metabolic pathway for β-oxidation [26]. Through β-oxidation IPPA is metabolized to iodobenzoic acid and its metabolite iodohippurate, and these are rapidly excreted from the kidneys with the iodine still attached, resulting in high image quality with low background by preventing the build-up of free radioiodide [27]. Coronary occlusion and reperfusion blunted the uptake of IPPA and prolonged the clearance, but permanent coronary occlusion decreased the uptake significantly and accelerated the clearance, indicating that the IPPA can be used to localize the area of myocardial ischemia and infarction [28]. However, still relatively fast rate of metabolism and clearance of IPPA precludes the clinical SPECT imaging, even in a rotating multi-detector SPECT system. For initial IPPA uptake imaging, acquisition time should be shortened to prevent progressive undersampling due to rapid count decrease from the myocardium, resulting in the deterioration of image quality, and dynamic SPECT study may be necessary for kinetic analysis of β-oxidation. For this purpose, dynamic SPECT with cadmium zinc-telluride (CZT) multi-detector might be the choice of data acquisition and analysis because of its high sensitivity [29].

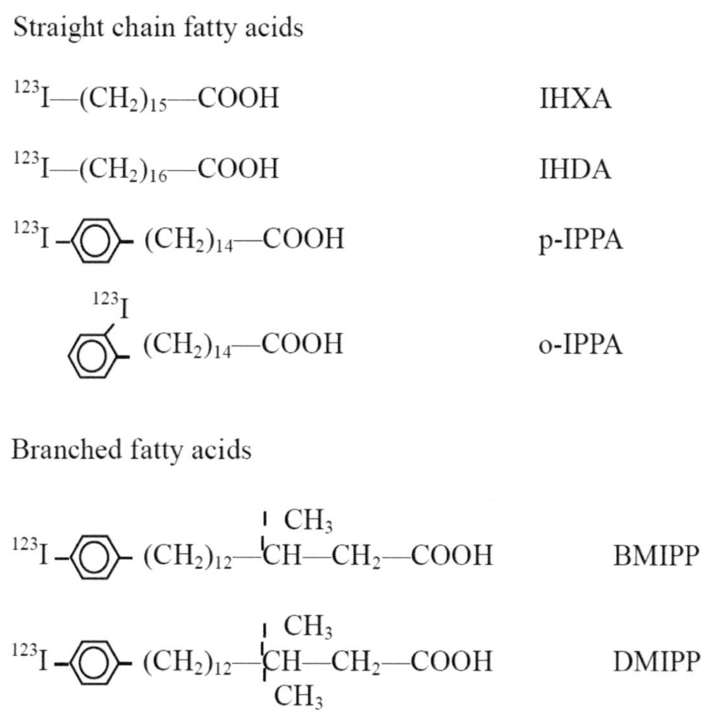

Figure 3. Iodinated fatty acids analogues for SPECT. BMIPP = β-methyl-iodophenyl pentadecanoic acid, DMIPP = dimethyl-iodophenyl pentadecanoic acid, IHDA = ^{123}I-heptadecanoic acid, IHXA =^{123}I-hexadecanoic acid, IPPA = iodophenyl pentadecanoic acid,

Accordingly, a new fatty acid tracer with more prolonged cardiac retention has been developed to improve quantitative image quality. For this purpose methyl branching was introduced at β-carbon position to slow myocardial clearance by inhibiting β-oxidation. Tow forms of iodine labeled modified fatty acids, 15-(p-iodophenyl)3-R, S-methylpentadecanoic acid (BMIPP) and 15-(p-iodophenyl)-3,3-dimethylpentadecanoic acid (DMIPP), has been developed [30,31]. In fasted rats, myocardial half-time of BMIPP and DMIPP are far longer, at 30-45 min and 6-7 hr, respectively, than that of IPPA (5-10 min) [31]. In human, DMIPP showed higher liver uptake than that of BMIPP (heart/liver ratio was 0.39 ± 0.05 and 1.00 ± 0.12, respectively: $p<0.001$), suggesting that BMIPP is more favorable cardiac SPECT agent [32]. Especially in Japan and some European countries, BMIPP has since been widely studied to investigate the clinical significance and basic properties. In Japan, ^{123}I-BMIPP has been used in daily clinical practice for nearly 2 decades since 1993.

4. Myocardial kinetic of ^{123}I-BMIPP (Fig 4)

After intravenous injection of ^{123}I-BMIPP, the tracer is delivered to myocardium depending on the regional flow and transported into myocardial cells via fatty acid translocase/CD36 involvement [10,11,13,16-18]. Once BMIPP is taken up by the myocyte, it will either back-diffuse to the plasma, accumulate in the lipid pool or undergo limited alpha and beta oxidation. Most of the BMIPP in the cytoplasm undergoes ATP dependent conversion to BMIPP-CoA and incorporated into triglyceride pool [31,33]. Canine study demonstrated that high first pass extraction (74%) within 30 sec of intracoronary BMIPP infusion, followed by a small fraction of washout (8.7% of infused BMIPP) for the next 30 min [34]. The washed out radioactiviy consist of backdiffused BMIPP (24% of all washed out radioactivity), α oxidation metabolite (27%), intermediate metabolites (33%), and full metabolite (16%), suggesting only small amount of BMIPP-CoA transported into mitochondria is metabolized by α oxidation (because first β oxidation is blocked by β-methyl branching), followed by β oxidation. The high uptake and low washout of the tracer indicates that BMIPP can be substantially considered as a metabolically trapped tracer like FDG.

Thirty minutes coronary occlusion and reperfusion was found to increase early back diffusion of nonmetabolized BMIPP from 25.1% to 34.7%, and in mild ischemia with 10 minutes occlusion, back diffusion of BMIPP was closely correlated with lactate production (marker of ischemic severity) [35]. Pharmacological intervention with etomoxir, one of the carnitine palmotoyltransferase I inhibitor that inhibits the transport of long chain lipids into the mitochondria, enhanced early washout of radioactivity until 8 minutes after injection due to increased back diffusion of BMIPP [36]. Dynamic SPECT in patients with coronary artery disease demonstrated that the BMIPP washout was observed early after BMIPP injection (2-6 min after injection) in the segments with stress induced thallium defects but not in the segments with normal thallium uptake and fixed thallium defects [37]. In patients with acute coronary syndrome, early dynamic BMIPP SPECT showed similar

BMIPP and thallium uptake, whereas conventional BMIPP images at 30 min demonstrated the discordant BMIPP uptake less than thallium [38]. These findings suggest that, in ischemic myocardium, initial myocardial distribution of BMIPP may represent blood flow, followed by back diffusion of free BMIPP which is not incorporated into triglyceride pool after conversion to BMIPP-CoA, resulting in discordant BMIPP uptake less than thallium on static images obtained 20-30 min after BMIPP injection.

In the first step of the common pathway of fatty acid metabolism, BMIPP also underwent ATP dependent conversion to BMIPP-CoA. Once BMIPP-CoA is synthesized, it is hardly back-diffused out of the cell and is retained within it [39,40]. Therefore, BMIPP myocardial retention may relate to the ATP level of the cells. Both in mouse myocardium treated with an electron transport uncoupler, dinitrophenol, which reduced intracellular ATP level without affecting acyl-CoA synthetase activity or CoA level, and in acutely damaged canine myocardium by coronary occlusion and reperfusion, BMIPP uptake was found to correlate with the tissue ATP levels [41,42]. Therefore, myocardial BMIPP uptake most likely reflects activation of BMIPP by CoA and indirectly reflects cellular ATP production resulting from fatty acid metabolism.

During acute phase of ischemia, reduced availability of oxygen suppresses β-oxidation and increases the proportion of fatty acid in the triglyceride pool. At this moment BMIPP may enter into this enlarged triglyceride pool. Accordingly, BMIPP uptake may possibly be increased in acute ischemia. Canine experiments with occlusion and reperfusion model showed higher BMIPP uptake than thallium (reverse mismatch) which is an opposite finding observed in clinical studies [43,44]. However, BMIPP uptake may change as a function of time after ischemia. A rat study with 20 min coronary occlusion and reperfusion demonstrated higher BMIPP uptake than thallium at 1 day after reperfusion but showed similar to or lower than thallium uptake at 5 day after reperfusion [45]. Another rat study with 20 min coronary occlusion and reperfusion revealed that increased BMIPP uptake in area at risk at 20 min and 1 day after reperfusion, followed by reduction of uptake at 3 to 7 days, though, recovered to normal level at 30 days after reperfusion [46]. By contrast, thallium uptake did not change throughout the 30 days observation period. As a result, higher BMIPP uptake than thallium in acute phase was inverted in subacute phase (discordant or mismatch BMIPP uptake less than thallium) and recovered to the similar uptake to that of thallium. After a transient ischemic insult, recovery of myocardial perfusion, metabolism and function may be temporally different. Although, delayed recovery of function after transient ischemia is well documented in the experimental and clinical setting as stunned myocardium, delayed recovery of regional metabolism or *metabolic stunning* which provide imprint prior ischemic event has been recognized recently. This delayed recovery of metabolism after quick recovery of perfusion provides a concept of *ischemic memory* imaging [47-50]. Thus BMIPP imaging during or after an episode of myocardial ischemia might provide crucial insights into pathophysiology of coronary artery disease over perfusion imaging.

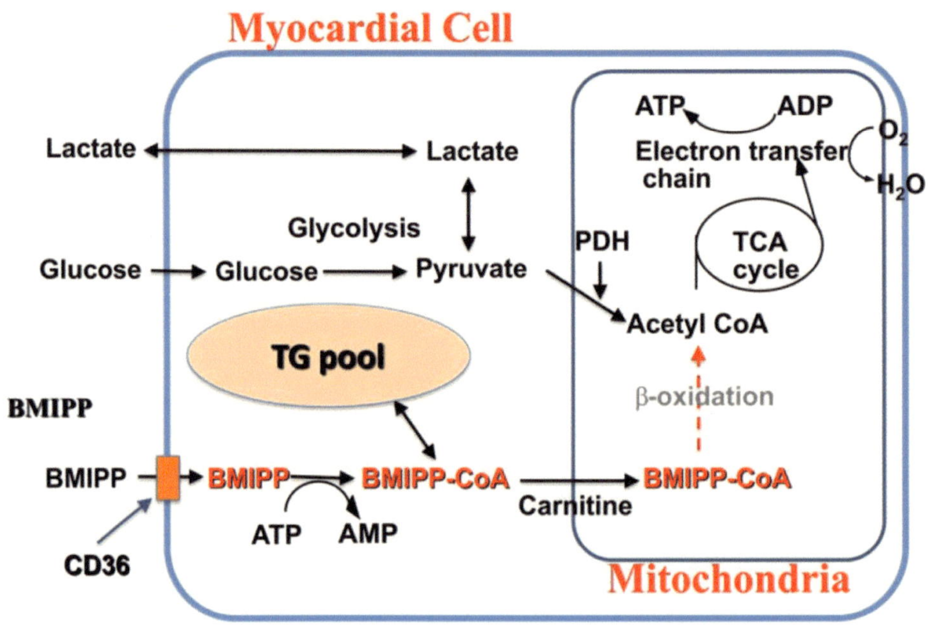

Figure 4. Schematic presentation of ^{123}I-BMIPP metabolism in myocardium. Abbreviations: see Figure 1.

5. ^{123}I-BMIPP imaging in ischemic heart diseases

5.1. Acute myocardial infarction

Discrepant BMIPP uptake less than thallium has been reported initially in 17 out of 28 patients with acute myocardial infarction. Such discordant BMIPP uptake was observed more often in areas of acute than chronic phase of myocardial infarction (59% at <4 week versus 31% at >4 week after onset), and more often in areas supplied with revascularized than non-revascularized arteries (74% versus 28%, respectively). In addition, regional wall motion was more severely impaired in such perfusion-metabolic mismatching area [51]. In patients with acute myocardial infarction, BMIPP and ^{99m}Tc-MIBI SPECT at 4 to 10 days after thrombolysis demonstrated that the segments with more reduced BMIPP uptake than MIBI uptake (mismatching) showed either normal wall motion or demonstrated inotropic reserve during dobutamine stimulation [52]. In addition, several studies had demonstrated that areas of discordant BMIPP uptake less than perfusion tracers in acute or subacute stages of myocardial infarction showed improvement of wall motion abnormality on the subsequent follow-up periods [47,53-59]. These findings suggested that mismatch or discordant BMIPP uptake less than perfusion is indicative of jeopardized but viable myocardium and may correspond to stunned myocardium where functional abnormality is prolonged in association with sustained metabolic abnormalities (metabolically stunned myocardium) after perfusion recovery by successful reperfusion

http://dx.doi.org/10.5772/53548

procedures. Accordingly, the finding of mismatched BMIPP uptake less than perfusion tracers may be a predictor of functional recovery in acute myocardial infarction. For the evaluation of area at risk in acute myocardial infarction, BMIPP imaging in subacute phase is valuable. BMIPP defect size in subacute phase of myocardial infarction correlated well with the risk area revealed by contrast ventriculography or echocardiography [47,60], and the area with BMIPP reduction 1 week after the onset of myocardial infarction corresponded well to the area with perfusion defect which was demonstrated before revascularization therapy at admission [61]. These observations holds the concept of "*ischemic memory imaging*" because BMIPP imaging obtained in subacute phase of myocardial infarction reflects prior ischemic damage or metabolically stunned myocardium even after the restoration of perfusion abnormality [47-49]. Therefore, BMIPP imaging may contribute to improving the detection of culprit lesion of the small amount of acute myocardial infarction. In patients with non ST elevated and non serum creatinine kinase-MB elevated but increased cTnT level, BMIPP SPECT at subacute phase can detect culprit coronary lesions more sensitively than thallium [62].

Mismatched uptake of BMIPP less than thallium is not also an uncommon finding in chronic phase of myocardial infarction. In 26 patients with prior myocardial infarction (>4 week after onset) without revascularization therapy, resting BMIPP and exercise-redistribution thallium scintigraphies were studied. Sixty-seven % of the segments with discordant BMIPP uptake less than redistribution thallium showed reversible thallium defects, 21% showed fixed thallium defects and 12% showed normal thallium uptake, indicating that the myocardium with discordant BMIPP uptake less than redistribution thallium uptake were mostly exposed to stress induced ischemia [37]. In subacute to chronic phase of infraction (>2 week after onset), similar findings were reported, with most of the mismatched segments (22/27) is associated with reversible thallium defect [63].

5.2. Acute coronary syndrome and unstable angina pectoris

Because oxygen extraction by the myocardium is nearly complete, reduction of coronary flow against the myocardial oxygen demand evoke the metabolic switch from fatty acid oxidation to anaerobic glucose metabolism. Thus the BMIPP uptake might be suppressed in ischemia. In a study of 111 consecutive patients with acute chest pain without myocardial infarction, BMIPP SPECT at 2 days after the onset of chest pain showed regional abnormality in 74% of coronary abnormalities, while only 38% showed perfusion abnormality demonstrated by tetrofosmin within 24 hr after the onset of chest pain [64]. Recently, multicenter trial to evaluate the performance of BMIPP to detect acute coronary syndromes in emergency department patients with chest pain was conducted in a total of 507 patients without history of prior myocardial infarction [65]. BMIPP imaging was performed within 30 hours of symptom cessation. Sensitivity of detecting acute coronary syndrome increased from 43% in clinical diagnosis to 73% in BMIPP imaging alone. Both negative and positive predictive values of a clinical diagnosis alone increased significantly when combined BMIPP imaging from 62% to 83% and 41% to 58%, respectively.

These findings indicates that BMIPP imaging can detect prolonged metabolic abnormality or stunning in patients with acute chest pain up to 2 days after cessation of symptom.

In patients with unstable angina, discordant BMIPP uptake less than thallium has also been observed frequently [66-69]. In patients with unstable angina without prior myocardial infarction, comparison of BMIPP image and stress thallium scan performed after stabilization of their condition demonstrated that BMIPP decrease was associated with stress perfusion abnormality in 44 of 57 (77%) segments and degree of BMIPP reduction correlated with the degree of perfusion abnormality at stress, degree of wall motion abnormality, and severity of coronary artery stenosis [66]. In another study in patients with unstable angina after medication and elimination of chest pain disclosed that patients with abnormal BMIPP uptake had more severe coronary artery stenosis and more collateral opacification than patients without BMIPP abnormality. In addition, revascularization was performed in 82% of patients with abnormal BMIPP images, while in only 22% of patients with normal BMIPP images, accordingly, BMIPP imaging may be helpful in decision-making regarding interventional treatment [68]. These findings indicate that reduced BMIPP uptake in patients with unstable angina may represent persistent metabolic abnormality reflecting prior severe ischemia or repetitive ischemic insults, thus the concept of ischemic memory imaging could be extended and applied to these patients population. In other words, BMIPP imaging could extend time window for detecting previous ischemic event after the resolution of perfusion abnormality.

5.3. Chronic stable coronary artery disease

In chronic stable coronary artery disease even without history of myocardial infarction, discordant BMIPP uptake less than perfusion tracer is also a common finding. Comparison of BMIPP and stress-reinjection thallium SPECT in 45 patients with chronic coronary artery disease demonstrated that most of the segments (118/124) with discordant BMIPP uptake less than reinjection-thallium were associated with demand ischemia indicated by reversible thallium defects [70]. When reversible thallium defects were analyzed, approximately half of the segments evidenced discordant BMIPP uptake less than reinjection thallium. On the other hand, around 80% of the segments with fixed thallium defects demonstrated concordant reduction of both tracers, suggesting myocardium with reduced or poor viability has metabolic abnormality similar to the degree of resting perfusion abnormality. When reversible thallium defects were analyzed with respect to the evidence of discordant BMIPP uptake less than thallium and regional wall motion abnormality, wall motion was more severely impaired in the segments with discordant BMIPP uptake less than thallium than those without such discordance in both subset of patients with and without old myocardial infarction. However, severity of coronary artery stenosis was similar in the vascular teritory with discordant BMIPP uptake less than reinjection thallium and those without such discordance. Comparison of BMIPP and stress-redistribution-reinjection thallium imaging in 55 patients with stable coronary artery disease revealed that discordant BMIPP uptake less than thallium was observed in only 37% of the segments with thallium redistribution after exercise, on the contrary, such discordance was observed in 82% of the segments with no redistribution but new fill-in after thallium reinjection [71]. In addition, such discordance was observed in only 19% of the segments with fixed defects. Previous studies with stress-redistribution-reinjection thallium demonstrated that the myocardium with new fill-in after thallium reinjection is characterized as severely ischemic but viable myocardium with frequent wall motion abnormalities that may recover after revascularization [72,73]. Accordingly, these observation may indicate that discordant BMIPP uptake less than thallium is suggestive of the myocardium jeopardized by more severe ischemia.

The concept of ischemic memory imaging of BMIPP has been tested in 32 patients with exercise-induced ischemia on thallium SPECT. BMIPP imaging at rest within 30 hrs of ischemia, which was induced and confirmed by exercise thallium SPECT, revealed reduction of BMIPP uptake corresponding to the ischemic area detected by stress thallium study in more than 90 % of patients [50]. Therefore, the authors concluded that BMIPP can identify sustained metabolic abnormality as a ischemic memory imaging at least until 30 hrs after stress induced ischemic episodes. This finding was complemented by the studies assessing glucose metabolism in patients undergoing exercise testing using FDG. Those have shown that a metabolic switch from fatty acid to glucose use occurs promptly when myocardial ischemia is induced during exercise and this metabolic switch to glucose may persist for 24hours, despite restoration of blood flow at rest [74,75].

Accumulated data in patients with chronic ischemic heart disease in Japan, however, demonstrated that reduced BMIPP uptake was frequently observed independent of prior radionuclide and ECG stress tests but related to severe ischemia and wall motion abnormality, raise the possibility that BMIPP reduction reflects the substrate shift from fatty acid to glucose as a results of repeated myocardial ischemia rather than reflecting the single episode of metabolic stunning. Myocardium exposed to repetitive ischemia or stunning is subsequently adapted metabolically (metabolic remodeling) into chronic ischemic myocardium, so called hibernation [76-78]. In hibernating myocardium, energy substrate is shifted from fatty acid to glucose, contractility is impaired but with recruitable inotropic reserve, and myocardial flow reserve is severely impaired. In relation to this issue, relationship between BMIPP uptake and absolute myocardial blood flow by PET was investigated in patients with chronic stable angina without previous myocardial infarction. The results demonstrated that rest myocardial blood flow was preserved independent of BMIPP uptake. However, hyperemic myocardial blood flow was decreased in the area with reduced BMIPP uptake, resulting in the severity of impaired myocardial flow reserve correlated to the reduction of BMIPP uptake [79]. Thus, reduced BMIPP uptake implies impaired myocardial flow reserve and may reflects adaptive substrate shifts or metabolic remodeling in hibernating myocardium. Representative case with stable angina pectoris who underwent BMIPP and thallium SPECT before and after coronary intervention (Fig 5).

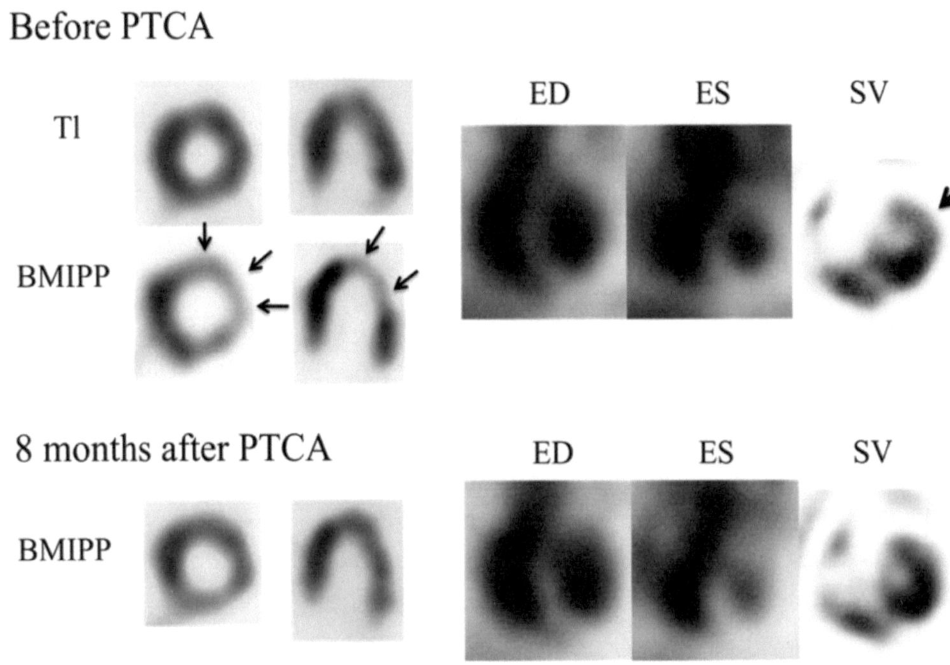

Figure 5. Short axis and horizontal long axis slices of ^{201}Tl, ^{123}I- BMIPP and gated blood pool images. The patient with angina pectoris underwent thallium and BMIPP SPECT. Discordant BMIPP uptake less than thallium in antero-lateral wall was observed (arrows). Gated blood pool scintigraphy demonstrated mild hypokinesis in antero-lateral wall. Stroke volume image showed reduced stroke volume in anterolateral wall (arrow). Coronary angiography showed severe stenosis of the first diagonal brunch of the left anterior descending coronary artery. Coronary angioplasty was successfully performed and BMIPP uptake and wall motion abnormality improved 8 month later. The discordant BMIPP uptake less than thallium depicted the dysfunctional but viable myocardium or hibernating myocardium in anterolateral wall. ED = end-diastolic, ES = end-systolic, PTCA = percutaneous transluminal coronary angioplasty, SV = stroke volume

5.4. Detection of coronary artery disease

Meta-analysis for the assessment of diagnostic accuracy of BMIPP imaging for the detection of coronary artery disease was conducted with 7 studies between 1995 and 2004 [80]. A total of 528 patients with a high prevalence of coronary artery disease who underwent both BMIPP imaging and coronary angiography were analyzed using a random-effects model. The overall sensitivity and specificity were 78% (95% confidence interval, 73% to 81%) and 84% (95% confidence interval, 77% to 89%). The summary receiver operating characteristic curve analysis showed that the area under the curve was 0.91 (SE, 0.020), and the Q* index was 0.84 (SE, 0.022), indicating excellent diagnostic accuracy. This diagnostic performance is comparable with stress myocardial perfusion SPECT reported by meta-analysis; a sensitivity and specificity of 88% and 73%, respectively [81]. Thus, stress SPECT imaging is a more sensitive test, whereas BMIPP imaging is a more specific test. Unlike stress myocardial perfusion imaging, BMIPP imaging is obtained without the use of exercise or pharmacologic agents. Therefore, BMIPP imaging at rest may be an alternative imaging modality for those

http://dx.doi.org/10.5772/53548

who are unable to perform adequate exercise testing or pharmacologic stress myocardial perfusion imaging, such as those presenting with acute chest pain and patients with end stage renal disease with hemodialysis.

5.5. Myocardial viability assessment and prediction of functional recovery

Improvement of regional or global systolic function can be achieved if revascularization of viable myocardium is successfully performed. Therefore, assessment of residual myocardial viability in the setting of dysfunctional myocardium due to significant coronary artery disease is a key issue in making clinical decisions with respect to revascularization procedures. In this respect, stress myocardial perfusion SPECT has been extensively investigated. The hallmarks of myocardial viability supplied by a stenosed or occluded coronary artery are the perfusion defect with thallium redistribution on stress-redistribution or rest-redistribution images, fill-in of thallium, setamibi, and tetrofosmin after reinjection, or significant uptake on resting or reinjection images (usually more than 50-60% uptake of normal area). However, the ability of perfusion tracers to differentiate viable from non-viable myocardium is not completely satisfactory as evidenced by recent viability studies using perfusion tracers [82-84]. In terms of the hallmark of viability in BMIPP imaging, there are several substantial evidences that discordant BMIPP uptake less than perfusion tracers is a marker of viability; 1) as previously described, such mismatch is associated with ischemic myocardium as evidenced by stress perfusion studies, 2) increased FDG uptake was observed in areas with discordant BMIPP uptake less than thallium and higher oxidative metabolism by ^{11}C-acetate PET was observed in mismatched area than the area with concordant reduction of BMIPP and perfusion [85], 3) myocardial areas with BMIPP uptake less than sestamibi were more likely to have a positive response to dobutamine than areas with matched defect [86,87], 4) histologic examination in patients with bypass surgery demonstrated that BMIPP uptake reduction against % fibrosis looked biphasic, with steep reduction of BMIPP uptake within 20% of fibrosis, although, thallium uptake reduction correlated linearly to % fibrosis, implying the areas with discordant BMIPP uptake less than thallium had less than 20% fibrosis [88].

Functional recovery after revascularization has been investigated in relation to BMIPP uptake abnormality in patients with chronic coronary artery disease. Discordant BMIPP uptake less than thallium could predict functional recovery after revascularization more precisely than exercise-reinjection thallium study. In addition, the extent of discordance were a good predictor of global ejection fraction improvement after revascularization [89]. Similarly, area with discordant BMIPP uptake less than sestamibi measured by quantitative analysis was highly predictive of improvement of ejection fraction, wall motion and free fatty acid utilization after revascularization [87]. Interestingly, the comparison of FDG, BMIPP, and sestamibi uptake in patients with old myocardial infarction and stable ischemic regional wall motion abnormalities demonstrated that extent of discordant BMIPP uptake less than FDG uptake before revascularization highly correlated with ejection fraction improvement after revascularization ($r = 0.74$) and also the extent of discordant BMIPP uptake less than sestamibi correlated significantly with ejection fraction improvement ($r = 0.50$). However, no significant correlation was observed between the area with discordant FDG uptake more than sestamib and ejection fraction recovery [90]. The results are quite intuitive because, in ischemic and viable myocardium, substrate shift from fatty acid to glucose would take place, hence, mismatch of FDG and BMIPP uptake should be prominent but mismatch between BMIPP and sestamibi might be modest. These data suggest that discordant BMIPP uptake less than perfusion may represent reversible ischemic myocardial injury or hibernating myocardium and that the regional and global dysfunction will improve after revascularization in patients with chronic stable coronary artery disease. Metabolic stunning is also a good marker of functional recovery. In acute myocardial infarction with emergency revascularization, BMIPP and tetrofosmin mismatch around 1 week after the revascularization predicted recovery of ejection fraction and wall motion 3 month later [91,92].

5.6. Risk stratification and prediction of the prognosis

Assessment of prognostic value of BMIPP imaging over perfusion tracers in patients with coronary artery disease is a matter of clinical importance. The initial study for the assessment of prognostic implications of BMIPP imaging was conducted in 50 consecutive patients with myocardial infarction with a mean follow up period of 23 months [93]. During the follow-up period, 9 patients had cardiac events; 8 of the 9 patients with cardiac events showed discordant BMIPP uptake less than reinjection thallium, whereas only 20 of 41 patients without cardiac events showed such mismatch. When all the clinical and radionuclide variables were analyzed by Cox regression analysis, presence of discordant BMIPP uptake was the best, and an independent, predictor of future cardiac events followed by the number of coronary artery stenosis. BMIPP and thallium imaging performed within 1 month of acute myocardial infarction demonstrated that impaired BMIPP uptake and mismatched BMIPP uptake less than thallium are related to a high probability of fatal and non-fatal cardiac events [94] and the defect score of BMIPP and mismatched BMIPP uptake less than thallium provided incremental predictive value for future cardiac events [95,96].

In the patients with chronic stage of myocardial infarction, clinical value of BMIPP imaging for predicting prognosis is also demonstrated. BMIPP imaging performed before revascularization in 76 patients with chronic stable ischemia (including 61 patients with myocardial infarction after at least 3 month of onset) with left ventricular dysfunction has been analyzed [97]. Patients with large amount of discordant BMIPP uptake less than thallium demonstrated greater ejection fraction improvement after revascularization and, interestingly, showed significantly better event free survival than patients with small amount or no perfusion and metabolic mismatch. These data indicate that patients with significant amount of discordant BMIPP uptake less than thallium may benefit from revascularization.

In chronic coronary artery disease without old myocardial infarction, value of BMIPP imaging for risk stratification has been also demonstrated. In 270 patients, BMIPP defect score was analyzed with respect to cardiac event during a median follow-up of 3.9 years [98]. Kaplan-Meier survival estimates revealed that patients with a summed BMIPP defect score lower than 5 showed a better prognosis than the patients with more defect of BMIPP (a hard event-free survival rate at 3 years: 98% vs 93% ($P = 0.03$), all event-free survival rate at 3

http://dx.doi.org/10.5772/53548

years: 92% vs 80% (P = 0.0003), respectively). More importantly, BMIPP was able to select a high-risk subgroup among patients with diabetes mellitus as well as non-diabetic patients, with 41% event rate in diabetic patients with BMIPP defect score 5 or more but only 4% event rate in non-diabetic patients with BMIPP defect score lower than 5.

One of the strength of BMIPP imaging in daily clinical use is its simplicity since it offers metabolic information without stress procedure. It is a matter of great interest whether resting BMIPP imaging offers complementary or additional prognostic information to that provided conventional stress perfusion imaging. One hundred and sity-seven consecutive patients with angina pectoris but without prior myocardial infarction who had undergone both BMIPP and stress thallium imaging were followed up for 48 months [99]. For overall cardiac events (5 hard and 29 soft events), multivariate Cox's analysis revealed that reduced BMIPP uptake, stress perfusion score, diabetes, and left ventricular ejection fraction were the significant predictors. No hard event was observed with normal BMIPP uptake, whereas 2 patients with nearly normal stress perfusion with impaired BMIPP uptake had a hard event. The authors concluded that resting BMIPP imaging may provide significant prognostic information independent of stress myocardial perfusion imaging.

Recently meta-analysis on the prognostic value of BMIPP imaging in acute coronary syndrome, acute myocardial infarction, and stable coronary artery disease was reported [100]. In 3 studies involving 541 patients with suspected acute coronary syndrome who were excluded for acute myocardial infarction, an abnormal finding on BMIPP imaging significantly associated with future hard cardiac events, defined as cardiac death and non-fatal myocardial infarction. The negative predictive value of BMIPP imaging for future hard and soft events were 98.9% and 92.3% over 3.5 years, respectively. In 6 studies which comprised 607 patients with acute myocardial infarction, larger defect on BMIPP imaging was significantly associated with cardiac death and hard events with relative risk of 2.81 and 3.87, respectively. Two studies included 166 patients with stable coronary artery disease who underwent elective revascularization. Both studies evaluated the prognostic value of mismatched BMIPP uptake less than perfusion, and showed contrasting results depending on the timing of BMIPP imaging to relative to revascularization. The presence of mismatched myocardium before revascularization, which suggested a jeopardized but viable myocardium, is associated with fewer events if patients undergo successful revascularization. However, the mismatch occurs after revascularization, indicating residual ischemia, the more hard events occur.

5.7. Chronic kidney disease

In chronic kidney disease (CKD), cardiovascular disease accounts for most of the morbidity and mortality in both pre-dialysis and after the onset of end stage renal disease. Stress myocardial perfusion imaging has become increasingly recognized as a powerful prognostic tool for cardiovascular outcomes in patents with known or suspected coronary artery disease. Abnormal stress myocardial perfusion scan is more common in patients with CKD and stress perfusion imaging is confirmed as a powerful tool for predicting outcomes across entire spectrum of renal dysfunction. At the same time, presence of CKD itself added prognostic value to perfusion imaging [101]. While stress perfusion imaging is valuable method to assess coronary artery disease, stress test may not be suitable for substantial number of CKD patients, especially in end stage renal disease. Because an inability to exercise enough due to multiple comorbidity including obesity, arthritis, and deconditioning etc, and suboptimal vasodilator stress testing due to an incomplete vasodilator response due to endothelial dysfunction. In this context, BMIPP imaging can be performed safely and effectively at rest to detect metabolic alteration due to ischemia without stress testing.

In addition to the high prevalence of coronary artery disease in patients with CKD, several sequelae of renal failure also contribute to left ventricular metabolic remodeling, so-called uremic cardiomyopathy. In this condition, myocyte capillary mismatch, with diminished vascular supply relative to the number and volume of functioning myocytes is observed [102,103]. These epicardial and microvascular disorder should induce ischemia when cardiac demand increases. For the detection of coronary artery disease in asymptomatic patients undergoing hemodialysis, dual isotope SPECT with thallium and BMIPP was investigated [104]. Significant coronary stenosis (>75%) was found in 72% of patients (93/130). When a BMIPP summed score of 6 or more was defined as abnormal, sensitivity, specificity, and accuracy for detecting coronary artery disease by BMIPP SPECT were 98.0%, 65.6%, and 90.0%, respectively. For the assessment of prognostic value of BMIPP in patients with hemodialysis, 318 asymptomatic patients without prior myocardial infarction underwent dual isotope SPECT with thallium and BMIPP [105]. During a mean follow up period of 3.6 ± 1.0 years, 50 died of cardiac event. Kaplan-Meier analysis showed that the cardiac death-free survival rates at 3 years were 61% and 98% in patients with BMIPP summed scores of >12 and <12, respectively. When the cutoff value of BMIPP–Tl mismatch score, a marker of ischemia, was determined to be 7, the sensitivity and specificity of BMIPP–Tl mismatch for predicting cardiac death were 86% and 88%, respectively. Kaplan-Meier survival estimates revealed that the event-free rates of cardiac death at 3 years were 53% in patients with BMIPP–Tl mismatch of > 7, whereas 96% in patients with BMIPP–Tl mismatch < 7. These finding suggested that significantly impaired myocardial fatty acid metabolism detected by BMIPP SPECT might predict the occurrence of cardiac death in asymptomatic hemodialysis patients. In addition, in patients with hemodialysis and complete coronary revascularization, BMIPP imaging abnormality and BMIPP thallium mismatch can also predict cardiac death [106]. Further more, prospectively enrolled 155 patients receiving hemodialysis after angiography had confirmed the absence of obstructive coronary lesions were examined by BMIPP SPECT [107]. During a mean follow-up of 5.1 years, 42 patients died of cardiac events. Stepwise Cox hazard analysis demonstrated that cardiac death asscociated with reduced BMIPP uptake and increased insulin resistance. Thus, impaired myocardial fatty acid metabolism and insulin resistance may be associated with cardiac death among hemodialysis patients without obstructive coronary artery disease.

Accordingly, in patients with high risk CKD, BMIPP imaging at rest is highly valuable in terms of the assessment of the myocardial metabolic abnormality, stratifying the patient's risk, and predicting cardiac death.

http://dx.doi.org/10.5772/53548

6. Summary and conclusions

In normal condition approximately two-thirds or more of the total energy produced by myocardium is derived from fatty acid oxidation and myocardial substrates may change significantly in various pathological conditions such as ischemia. Accordingly, many fatty acid tracers for SPECT imaging have been introduced. Until now, ^{123}I-BMIPP, one of the methyl branched fatty acid analogues, is the only approved fatty acid tracer for daily clinical use. The concept of BMIPP imaging is metabolic trapping, like FDG, by inhibiting β-oxidation by introducing methyl branching at β-carbon position. Myocardial BMIPP uptake more likely reflects activation of BMIPP into BMIPP-CoA with consumption of ATP, thus the uptake indirectly reflects cellular ATP production by fatty acid metabolism. Under the condition of ischemia, the reduction of BMIPP uptake is observed by reflecting the reduction of ATP production due to depressed oxidative fatty acid metabolism and substrate shift from fatty acids to glucose. Reduced uptake of BMIPP at rest is often observed in ischemic myocardium independent of the uptake of perfusion tracers, that is, discordant or mismatched BMIPP uptake less than perfusion tracers. Through comparison with perfusion, BMIPP image can detect previous myocardial ischemia as an ischemic memory imaging (stunned myocardium or status of metabolic stunning) and viable but chronically dysfunctional myocardium (hibernating myocardium or status of metabolic remodeling). In addition, BMIPP image may offer incremental prognostic information in ischemic heart diseases. Through the basic and clinical studies, it has become clear that BMIPP imaging has a high potential utility in the entire spectrum of ischemic heart diseases in evaluating the patients with acute chest pain, acute myocardial infarction, unstable angina pectoris, chronic stable coronary artery diseases, in terms of diagnosis, risk stratification, and also for the prediction of prognosis.

Author details

Junichi Taki[1], Ichiro Matsunari[2], Hiroshi Wakabayashi[1], Anri Inaki[1] and Seigo Kinuya[1]

1 Department of Nuclear Medicine, Kanazawa University Hospital, Kanazawa, Japan

2 Medical & Pharmacological Research Center Foundation, Hakui, Japan

References

[1] Taki J, Matsunari I. Metabolic imaging using SPECT. Eur J Nucl Med Mol Imaging. 2007 Jun;34 Suppl 1:S34-48.

[2] Tamaki N, Morita K, Kawai Y. The Japanese experience with metabolic imaging in the clinical setting. J Nucl Cardiol. 2007;14(3 Suppl):S145-52.

[3] Goodwin GW, Taegtmeyer H. Improved energy homeostasis of the heart in the metabolic state of exercise. Am J Physiol Heart Circ Physiol. 2000;279:H1490–H1501.

[4] Korvald C, Elvenes OP, Myrmel T. Myocardial substrate metabolism influences left ventricular energetics in vivo. Am J Physiol Heart Circ Physiol. 2000; 278(4):H1345-51.

[5] Liedtke AJ. Alterations of carbohydrate and lipid metabolism in the acutely ischemic heart. Prog Cardiovasc Dis 1981;23:321-36

[6] Camici P, Ferrannini E and Opie LH. Myocardial metabolism in ischemic heart disease: basic principles and application to imaging by positron emission tomography. Prog Cardiovasc Dis 1989;32:217-38

[7] Lopaschuk GD, Collins-Nakai RL, Itoi T. Developmental changes in energy substrate use by the heart. Cardiovascular Research. 1992;26(12):1172–80.

[8] Hwang EH, Yamashita A, Takemori H, Taki J, Nakajima K, Bunko H, et al. Absent myocardial I-123 BMIPP uptake in a family. Ann Nucl Med 1996;10:445-8

[9] Hashimoto J, Koseki S, Kinoshita F, Kubo A, Iwanaga S, Mitamura H, et al. Absent myocardial accumulation of two different radioiodinated pentadecanoic acids. Ann Nucl Med 1998;12:43-6

[10] Tanaka T, Okamoto F, Sohmiya K and Kawamura K. Lack of myocardial iodine-123 15-(p-iodiphenyl)-3-R,S-methylpentadecanoic acid (BMIPP) uptake and CD36 abnormality--CD36 deficiency and hypertrophic cardiomyopathy. Jpn Circ J 1997;61:724-5

[11] Hwang EH, Taki J, Yasue S, Fujimoto M, Taniguchi M, Matsunari I, et al. Absent myocardial iodine-123-BMIPP uptake and platelet/monocyte CD36 deficiency. J Nucl Med 1998;39:1681-4

[12] Yoshizumi T, Nozaki S, Fukuchi K, Yamasaki K, Fukuchi T, Maruyama T, et al. Pharmacokinetics and metabolism of 123I-BMIPP fatty acid analog in healthy and CD36-deficient subjects. J Nucl Med 2000;41:1134-8

[13] Watanabe K, Ohta Y, Toba K, Ogawa Y, Hanawa H, Hirokawa Y, et al. Myocardial CD36 expression and fatty acid accumulation in patients with type I and II CD36 deficiency. Ann Nucl Med 1998;12:261-6

[14] Fukuchi K, Nozaki S, Yoshizumi T, Hasegawa S, Uehara T, Nakagawa T, et al. Enhanced myocardial glucose use in patients with a deficiency in long-chain fatty acid transport (CD36 deficiency). J Nucl Med 1999;40:239-43

[15] Kudoh T, Tamaki N, Magata Y, Konishi J, Nohara R, Iwasaki A, et al. Metabolism substrate with negative myocardial uptake of iodine-123-BMIPP. J Nucl Med 1997;38:548-53

[16] Nozaki S, Tanaka T, Yamashita S, Sohmiya K, Yoshizumi T, Okamoto F, et al. CD36 mediates long-chain fatty acid transport in human myocardium: complete myocar-

dial accumulation defect of radiolabeled long-chain fatty acid analog in subjects with CD36 deficiency. Mol Cell Biochem 1999;192:129-35

[17] Tanaka T, Nakata T, Oka T, Ogawa T, Okamoto F, Kusaka Y, et al. Defect in human myocardial long-chain fatty acid uptake is caused by FAT/CD36 mutations. J Lipid Res 2001;42:751-9

[18] Brinkmann JF, Abumrad NA, Ibrahimi A, van der Vusse GJ and Glatz JF. New insights into long-chain fatty acid uptake by heart muscle: a crucial role for fatty acid translocase/CD36. Biochem J 2002;367:561-70

[19] Robinson GD, Jr. and Lee AW. Radioiodinated fatty acids for heart imaging: iodine monochloride addition compared with iodide replacement labeling. J Nucl Med 1975;16:17-21

[20] Poe ND, Robinson GD, Jr., Graham LS and MacDonald NS. Experimental basis of myocardial imaging with 123I-labeled hexadecenoic acid. J Nucl Med 1976;17:1077-82

[21] Poe ND, Robinson GD, Jr., Zielinski FW, Cabeen WR, Jr., Smith JW and Gomes AS. Myocardial imaging with 123I-hexadecenoic acid. Radiology 1977;124:419-24

[22] Visser FC, van Eenige MJ, Westera G, Den Hollander W, Duwel CM, van der Wall EE, et al. Metabolic fate of radioiodinated heptadecanoic acid in the normal canine heart. Circulation 1985;72:565-71

[23] Freundlieb C, Hock A, Vyska K, Feinendegen LE, Machulla HJ and Stocklin G. Myocardial imaging and metabolic studies with [17-123I]iodoheptadecanoic acid. J Nucl Med 1980;21:1043-50

[24] Machulla HJ, Marsmann M and Dutschka K. Biochemical concept and synthesis of a radioiodinated phenylfatty acid for in vivo metabolic studies of the myocardium. Eur J Nucl Med 1980;5:171-3

[25] Reske SN, Sauer W, Machulla HJ and Winkler C. 15(p-[123I]Iodophenyl)pentadecanoic acid as tracer of lipid metabolism: comparison with [1-14C]palmitic acid in murine tissues. J Nucl Med 1984;25:1335-42

[26] Caldwell JH, Martin GV, Link JM, Krohn KA and Bassingthwaighte JB. Iodophenylpentadecanoic acid-myocardial blood flow relationship during maximal exercise with coronary occlusion. J Nucl Med 1990;31:99-105

[27] Ercan M, Senekowitsch R, Bauer R, Reidel G, Kriegel H and Pabst HW. In vivo and in vitro studies with omega-[rho-123I-phenyl]-pentadecanoic acid in rats. Int J Appl Radiat Isot 1983;34:1519-24

[28] Rellas JS, Corbett JR, Kulkarni P, Morgan C, Devous MD, Sr., Buja LM, et al. Iodine-123 phenylpentadecanoic acid: detection of acute myocardial infarction and injury in dogs using an iodinated fatty acid and single-photon emission tomography. Am J Cardiol 1983;52:1326-32

[29] Garcia EV. Quantitative Nuclear Cardiology: we are almost there! J Nucl Cardiol. 2012 ;19(3):424-37.

[30] Goodman MM, Kirsch G and Knapp FF, Jr. Synthesis and evaluation of radioiodinated terminal p-iodophenyl-substituted alpha- and beta-methyl-branched fatty acids. J Med Chem 1984;27:390-7

[31] Knapp FF, Jr., Ambrose KR and Goodman MM. New radioiodinated methyl-branched fatty acids for cardiac studies. Eur J Nucl Med 1986;12 Suppl:S39-44

[32] Sloof GW, Visser FC, van Lingen A, Bax JJ, Eersels J, Teule GJ, et al. Evaluation of heart-to-organ ratios of 123I-BMIPP and the dimethyl-substituted 123I-DMIPP fatty acid analogue in humans. Nucl Med Commun 1997;18:1065-70

[33] Ambrose KR, Owen BA, Goodman MM and Knapp FF, Jr. Evaluation of the metabolism in rat hearts of two new radioiodinated 3-methyl-branched fatty acid myocardial imaging agents. Eur J Nucl Med 1987;12:486-91

[34] Fujibayashi Y, Nohara R, Hosokawa R, Okuda K, Yonekura Y, Tamaki N, et al. Metabolism and kinetics of iodine-123-BMIPP in canine myocardium. J Nucl Med 1996;37:757-61

[35] Hosokawa R, Nohara R, Fujibayashi Y, Okuda K, Ogino M, Hata T, et al. Myocardial kinetics of iodine-123-BMIPP in canine myocardium after regional ischemia and reperfusion: implications for clinical SPECT. J Nucl Med 1997;38:1857-63

[36] Hosokawa R, Nohara R, Fujibayashi Y, Okuda K, Ogino M, Hata T, et al. Metabolic fate of iodine-123-BMIPP in canine myocardium after administration of etomoxir. J Nucl Med 1996;37:1836-40

[37] Matsunari I, Saga T, Taki J, Akashi Y, Hirai J, Wakasugi T, et al. Kinetics of iodine-123-BMIPP in patients with prior myocardial infarction: assessment with dynamic rest and stress images compared with stress thallium-201 SPECT. J Nucl Med 1994;35:1279-85

[38] Kobayashi H, Kusakabe K, Momose M, Okawa T, Inoue S, Iguchi N, et al. Evaluation of myocardial perfusion and fatty acid uptake using a single injection of iodine-123-BMIPP in patients with acute coronary syndromes. J Nucl Med 1998;39:1117-22

[39] Fox KA, Abendschein DR, Ambos HD, Sobel BE and Bergmann SR. Efflux of metabolized and nonmetabolized fatty acid from canine myocardium. Implications for quantifying myocardial metabolism tomographically. Circ Res 1985;57:232-43

[40] Duwel CM, Visser FC, van Eenige MJ and Roos JP. Variables of myocardial backdiffusion, determined with 17-iodo-131 heptadecanoic acid in the normal dog heart. Mol Cell Biochem 1989;88:191-4

[41] Fujibayashi Y, Yonekura Y, Takemura Y, Wada K, Matsumoto K, Tamaki N, et al. Myocardial accumulation of iodinated beta-methyl-branched fatty acid analogue, io-

dine-125-15-(p-iodophenyl)-3-(R,S)methylpentadecanoic acid (BMIPP), in relation to ATP concentration. J Nucl Med 1990;31:1818-22

[42] Nohara R, Okuda K, Ogino M, Hosokawa R, Tamaki N, Konishi J, et al. Evaluation of myocardial viability with iodine-123-BMIPP in a canine model. J Nucl Med 1996;37:1403-7

[43] Miller DD, Gill JB, Livni E, Elmaleh DR, Aretz T, Boucher CA, et al. Fatty acid analogue accumulation: a marker of myocyte viability in ischemic-reperfused myocardium. Circ Res 1988;63:681-92

[44] Nishimura T, Sago M, Kihara K, Oka H, Shimonagata T, Katabuchi T, et al. Fatty acid myocardial imaging using 123I-beta-methyl-iodophenyl pentadecanoic acid (BMIPP): comparison of myocardial perfusion and fatty acid utilization in canine myocardial infarction (occlusion and reperfusion model). Eur J Nucl Med 1989;15:341-5

[45] Noriyasu K, Mabuchi M, Kuge Y, Morita K, Tsukamoto T, Kohya T, et al. Serial changes in BMIPP uptake in relation to thallium uptake in the rat myocardium after ischaemia. Eur J Nucl Med Mol Imaging 2003;30:1644-50

[46] Higuchi T, Taki J, Nakajima K, Kinuya S, Namura M and Tonami N. Time course of discordant BMIPP and thallium uptake after ischemia and reperfusion in a rat model. J Nucl Med 2005;46:172-5

[47] Naruse H, Arii T, Kondo T, Morita M, Ohyanagi M, Iwasaki T, et al. Clinical usefulness of iodine 123-labeled fatty acid imaging in patients with acute myocardial infarction. J Nucl Cardiol 1998;5:275-84

[48] Mochizuki T, Murase K, Higashino H, Miyagawa M, Sugawara Y, Kikuchi T, et al. Ischemic "memory image" in acute myocardial infarction of 123I-BMIPP after reperfusion therapy: a comparison with 99mTc-pyrophosphate and 201Tl dual-isotope SPECT. Ann Nucl Med 2002;16:563-8

[49] Tamaki N, Tadamura E, Kudoh T, Hattori N, Inubushi M and Konishi J. Recent advances in nuclear cardiology in the study of coronary artery disease. Ann Nucl Med 1997;11:55-66

[50] Dilsizian V, Bateman TM, Bergmann SR, Des Prez R, Magram MY, Goodbody AE, et al. Metabolic imaging with beta-methyl-p-[(123)I]-iodophenyl-pentadecanoic acid identifies ischemic memory after demand ischemia. Circulation 2005;112:2169-74

[51] Tamaki N, Kawamoto M, Yonekura Y, Fujibayashi Y, Takahashi N, Konishi J, et al. Regional metabolic abnormality in relation to perfusion and wall motion in patients with myocardial infarction: assessment with emission tomography using an iodinated branched fatty acid analog. J Nucl Med 1992;33:659-67

[52] Franken PR, De Geeter F, Dendale P, Demoor D, Block P and Bossuyt A. Abnormal free fatty acid uptake in subacute myocardial infarction after coronary thrombolysis: correlation with wall motion and inotropic reserve. J Nucl Med 1994;35:1758-65

[53] Ito T, Tanouchi J, Kato J, Morioka T, Nishino M, Iwai K, et al. Recovery of impaired left ventricular function in patients with acute myocardial infarction is predicted by the discordance in defect size on 123I-BMIPP and 201Tl SPET images. Eur J Nucl Med 1996;23:917-23

[54] Hashimoto A, Nakata T, Tsuchihashi K, Tanaka S, Fujimori K and Iimura O. Postischemic functional recovery and BMIPP uptake after primary percutaneous transluminal coronary angioplasty in acute myocardial infarction. Am J Cardiol 1996;77:25-30

[55] Franken PR, Dendale P, De Geeter F, Demoor D, Bossuyt A and Block P. Prediction of functional outcome after myocardial infarction using BMIPP and sestamibi scintigraphy. J Nucl Med 1996;37:718-22

[56] Nishimura T, Nishimura S, Kajiya T, Sugihara H, Kitahara K, Imai K, et al. Prediction of functional recovery and prognosis in patients with acute myocardial infarction by 123I-BMIPP and 201Tl myocardial single photon emission computed tomography: a multicenter trial. Ann Nucl Med 1998;12:237-48

[57] Hambye AS, Vervaet A, Dobbeleir A, Dendale P and Franken P. Prediction of functional outcome by quantification of sestamibi and BMIPP after acute myocardial infarction. Eur J Nucl Med 2000;27:1494-500

[58] Katsunuma E, Kurokawa S, Takahashi M, Fukuda N, Kurosawa T and Izumi T. Usefulness of BMIPP SPECT to evaluate myocardial viability, contractile reserve and coronary stenotic progression after reperfusion in acute myocardial infarction. Jpn Heart J 2001;42:435-49

[59] Seki H, Toyama T, Higuchi K, Kasama S, Ueda T, Seki R, et al. Prediction of functional improvement of ischemic myocardium with (123I-BMIPP SPECT and 99mTc-tetrofosmin SPECT imaging: a study of patients with large acute myocardial infarction and receiving revascularization therapy. Circ J 2005;69:311-9

[60] Furutani Y, Shiigi T, Nakamura Y, Nakamura H, Harada M, Yamamoto T, et al. Quantification of area at risk in acute myocardial infarction by tomographic imaging. J Nucl Med 1997;38:1875-82

[61] Kawai Y, Tsukamoto E, Nozaki Y, Kishino K, Kohya T and Tamaki N. Use of 123I-BMIPP single-photon emission tomography to estimate areas at risk following successful revascularization in patients with acute myocardial infarction. Eur J Nucl Med 1998;25:1390-5

[62] Fukushima Y, Toba M, Ishihara K, Mizumura S, Seino T, Tanaka K, et al. Usefulness of 201TlCl/ 123I-BMIPP dual-myocardial SPECT for patients with non-ST segment elevation myocardial infarction. Ann Nucl Med. 2008 ;22(5):363-9.

[63] Kawamoto M, Tamaki N, Yonekura Y, Tadamura E, Fujibayashi Y, Magata Y, et al. Combined study with I-123 fatty acid and thallium-201 to assess ischemic myocardi-

um: comparison with thallium redistribution and glucose metabolism. Ann Nucl Med 1994;8:47-54

[64] Kawai Y, Tsukamoto E, Nozaki Y, Morita K, Sakurai M and Tamaki N. Significance of reduced uptake of iodinated fatty acid analogue for the evaluation of patients with acute chest pain. J Am Coll Cardiol 2001;38:1888-94

[65] Kontos MC, Dilsizian V, Weiland F, DePuey G, Mahmarian JJ, Iskandrian AE, et al. Iodofiltic acid I 123 (BMIPP) fatty acid imaging improves initial diagnosis in emergency department patients with suspected acute coronary syndromes: a multicenter trial. J Am Coll Cardiol. 2010 ;56(4):290-9.

[66] Tateno M, Tamaki N, Yukihiro M, Kudoh T, Hattori N, Tadamura E, et al. Assessment of fatty acid uptake in ischemic heart disease without myocardial infarction. J Nucl Med 1996;37:1981-5

[67] Suzuki A, Takada Y, Nagasaka M, Kato R, Watanabe T, Shimokata K, et al. Comparison of resting beta-methyl-iodophenyl pentadecanoic acid (BMIPP) and thallium-201 tomography using quantitative polar maps in patients with unstable angina. Jpn Circ J 1997;61:133-8

[68] Takeishi Y, Fujiwara S, Atsumi H, Takahashi K, Sukekawa H and Tomoike H. Iodine-123-BMIPP imaging in unstable angina: a guide for interventional strategy. J Nucl Med 1997;38:1407-11

[69] Takeishi Y, Sukekawa H, Saito H, Nishimura S, Shibu T, Sasaki Y, et al. Impaired myocardial fatty acid metabolism detected by 123I-BMIPP in patients with unstable angina pectoris: comparison with perfusion imaging by 99mTc-sestamibi. Ann Nucl Med 1995;9:125-30

[70] Taki J, Nakajima K, Matsunari I, Bunko H, Takada S and Tonami N. Impairment of regional fatty acid uptake in relation to wall motion and thallium-201 uptake in ischaemic but viable myocardium: assessment with iodine-123-labelled beta-methyl-branched fatty acid. Eur J Nucl Med 1995;22:1385-92

[71] Matsunari I, Fujino S, Taki J, Senma J, Aoyama T, Wakasugi T, et al. Impaired fatty acid uptake in ischemic but viable myocardium identified by thallium-201 reinjection. Am Heart J 1996;131:458-65

[72] Tamaki N, Ohtani H, Yonekura Y, Nohara R, Kambara H, Kawai C, et al. Significance of fill-in after thallium-201 reinjection following delayed imaging: comparison with regional wall motion and angiographic findings. J Nucl Med 1990;31:1617-23

[73] Ohtani H, Tamaki N, Yonekura Y, Mohiuddin IH, Hirata K, Ban T, et al. Value of thallium-201 reinjection after delayed SPECT imaging for predicting reversible ischemia after coronary artery bypass grafting. Am J Cardiol 1990;66:394-9

[74] He ZX, Shi RF, Wu YJ, Tian YQ, Liu XJ, Wang SW, et al. Direct imaging of exercise-induced myocardial ischemia with fluorine-18-labeled deoxyglucose and Tc-99m-sestamibi in coronary artery disease. Circulation. 2003 ;108(10):1208-13.

[75] Dou KF, Yang MF, Yang YJ, Jain D, He ZX. Myocardial 18F-FDG uptake after exercise-induced myocardial ischemia in patients with coronary artery disease. J Nucl Med. 2008 ;49(12):1986-91.

[76] Kim SJ, Peppas A, Hong SK, Yang G, Huang Y, Diaz G, et al. Persistent stunning induces myocardial hibernation and protection: flow/function and metabolic mechanisms. Circ Res 2003;92:1233-9

[77] Camici PG and Rimoldi OE. Myocardial blood flow in patients with hibernating myocardium. Cardiovasc Res 2003;57:302-11

[78] Gerber BL, Vanoverschelde JL, Bol A, Michel C, Labar D, Wijns W, et al. Myocardial blood flow, glucose uptake, and recruitment of inotropic reserve in chronic left ventricular ischemic dysfunction. Implications for the pathophysiology of chronic myocardial hibernation. Circulation 1996;94:651-9

[79] Kageyama H, Morita K, Katoh C, Tsukamoto T, Noriyasu K, Mabuchi M, et al. Reduced 123I-BMIPP uptake implies decreased myocardial flow reserve in patients with chronic stable angina. Eur J Nucl Med Mol Imaging 2006;33:6-12

[80] Inaba Y, Bergmann SR. Diagnostic accuracy of beta-methyl-p-[123I]-iodophenyl-pentadecanoic acid (BMIPP) imaging: a meta-analysis. J Nucl Cardiol. 2008 May-Jun; 15(3):345-52.

[81] Heijenbrok-Kal MH, Fleischmann KE, Hunink MG. Stress echocardiography, stress single-photon-emission computed tomography and electron beam computed tomography for the assessment of coronary artery disease: a meta-analysis of diagnostic performance. Am Heart J. 2007 ;154(3):415-23

[82] Udelson JE, Bonow RO and Dilsizian V. The historical and conceptual evolution of radionuclide assessment of myocardial viability. J Nucl Cardiol 2004;11:318-34

[83] Srinivasan G, Kitsiou AN, Bacharach SL, Bartlett ML, Miller-Davis C and Dilsizian V. [18F]fluorodeoxyglucose single photon emission computed tomography: can it replace PET and thallium SPECT for the assessment of myocardial viability? Circulation 1998;97:843-50

[84] Bax JJ, Wijns W, Cornel JH, Visser FC, Boersma E, Fioretti PM. Accuracy of currently available techniques for prediction of functional recovery after revascularization in patients with left ventricular dysfunction due to chronic coronary artery disease: comparison of pooled data. J Am Coll Cardiol. 1997 ;30(6):1451-60

[85] Tamaki N, Tadamura E, Kawamoto M, Magata Y, Yonekura Y, Fujibayashi Y, et al. Decreased uptake of iodinated branched fatty acid analog indicates metabolic alterations in ischemic myocardium. J Nucl Med 1995;36:1974-80

[86] Hambye AS, Vaerenberg MM, Dobbeleir AA, Van den Heuvel PA and Franken PR. Abnormal BMIPP uptake in chronically dysfunctional myocardial segments: correlation with contractile response to low-dose dobutamine. J Nucl Med 1998;39:1845-50

[87] Hambye AS, Dobbeleir AA, Vervaet AM, Van den Heuvel PA and Franken PR. BMIPP imaging to improve the value of sestamibi scintigraphy for predicting functional outcome in severe chronic ischemic left ventricular dysfunction. J Nucl Med 1999;40:1468-76

[88] Kudoh T, Tadamura E, Tamaki N, Hattori N, Inubushi M, Kubo S, et al. Iodinated free fatty acid and 201T1 uptake in chronically hypoperfused myocardium: histologic correlation study. J Nucl Med 2000;41:293-6

[89] Taki J, Nakajima K, Matsunari I, Bunko H, Takata S, Kawasuji M, et al. Assessment of improvement of myocardial fatty acid uptake and function after revascularization using iodine-123-BMIPP. J Nucl Med 1997;38:1503-10

[90] Sato H, Iwasaki T, Toyama T, Kaneko Y, Inoue T, Endo K, et al. Prediction of functional recovery after revascularization in coronary artery disease using (18)F-FDG and (123)I-BMIPP SPECT. Chest 2000;117:65-72

[91] Biswas SK, Sarai M, Toyama H, Yamada A, Motoyama S, Harigaya H, et al. (123)I-BMIPP and (99m)Tc-TF discordance on myocardial scintigraphy and it's correlation with functional recovery following acute myocardial infarction: role of conventional echocardiography. Int J Cardiovasc Imaging. 2009 ;25(8):765-75.

[92] Biswas SK, Sarai M, Yamada A, Motoyama S, Harigaya H, Hara T, et al. Fatty acid metabolism and myocardial perfusion imaging for the evaluation of global left ventricular dysfunction following acute myocardial infarction: comparisons with echocardiography. Int J Cardiol. 2010;138(3):290-9.

[93] Tamaki N, Tadamura E, Kudoh T, Hattori N, Yonekura Y, Nohara R, et al. Prognostic value of iodine-123 labelled BMIPP fatty acid analogue imaging in patients with myocardial infarction. Eur J Nucl Med 1996;23:272-9

[94] Nakata T, Kobayashi T, Tamaki N, Kobayashi H, Wakabayashi T, Shimoshige S, et al. Prognostic value of impaired myocardial fatty acid uptake in patients with acute myocardial infarction. Nucl Med Commun 2000;21:897-906

[95] Nanasato M, Hirayama H, Ando A, Isobe S, Nonokawa M, Kinoshita Y, et al. Incremental predictive value of myocardial scintigraphy with 123I-BMIPP in patients with acute myocardial infarction treated with primary percutaneous coronary intervention. Eur J Nucl Med Mol Imaging 2004;31:1512-21

[96] Fukushima Y, Toba M, Ishihara K, Mizumura S, Seino T, Tanaka K, et al. Usefulness of 201TlCl/ 123I-BMIPP dual-myocardial SPECT for patients with non-ST segment elevation myocardial infarction. Ann Nucl Med. 2008 ;22(5):363-9.

[97] Fukuzawa S, Ozawa S, Shimada K, Sugioka J and Inagaki M. Prognostic values of perfusion-metabolic mismatch in Tl-201 and BMIPP scintigraphic imaging in patients with chronic coronary artery disease and left ventricular dysfunction undergoing revascularization. Ann Nucl Med 2002;16:109-15

[98] Chikamori T, Fujita H, Nanasato M, Toba M and Nishimura T. Prognostic value of I-123 15-(p-iodophenyl)-3-(R,S) methylpentadecanoic acid myocardial imaging in patients with known or suspected coronary artery disease. J Nucl Cardiol 2005;12:172-8

[99] Matsuki T, Tamaki N, Nakata T, Doi A, Takahashi H, Iwata M, et al. Prognostic value of fatty acid imaging in patients with angina pectoris without prior myocardial infarction: comparison with stress thallium imaging. Eur J Nucl Med Mol Imaging 2004;31:1585-91

[100] Inaba Y, Bergmann SR. Prognostic value of myocardial metabolic imaging with BMIPP in the spectrum of coronary artery disease: a systematic review. J Nucl Cardiol. 2010 ;17(1):61-70.

[101] Hakeem A, Bhatti S, Trevino AR, Samad Z, Chang SM. Non-invasive risk assessment in patients with chronic kidney disease. J Nucl Cardiol. 2011 ;18(3):472-85

[102] Dilsizian V, Fink JC. Deleterious effect of altered myocardial fatty acid metabolism in kidney disease. J Am Coll Cardiol. 2008 ;51(2):146-8

[103] Tyralla K, Amann K. Morphology of the heart and arteries in renal failure. Kidney Int Suppl. 2003 ;63(84):S80-3

[104] Nishimura M, Hashimoto T, Kobayashi H, Fukuda T, Okino K, Yamamoto N, et al. Myocardial scintigraphy using a fatty acid analogue detects coronary artery disease in hemodialysis patients. Kidney Int. 2004;66(2):811-9.

[105] Nishimura M, Tsukamoto K, Hasebe N, Tamaki N, Kikuchi K, Ono T. Prediction of cardiac death in hemodialysis patients by myocardial fatty acid imaging. J Am Coll Cardiol. 2008;51(2):139-45.

[106] Nishimura M, Tokoro T, Nishida M, Hashimoto T, Kobayashi H, Yamazaki S, et al. Myocardial fatty acid imaging identifies a group of hemodialysis patients at high risk for cardiac death after coronary revascularization. Kidney Int. 2008 ;74(4):513-20.

[107] Nishimura M, Tsukamoto K, Tamaki N, Kikuchi K, Iwamoto N, Ono T. Risk stratification for cardiac death in hemodialysis patients without obstructive coronary artery disease. Kidney Int. 2011;79(3):363-71.